Ayurved
and
Hepatic Disorders

Indian Medical Science Series No.121

Ayurved
and
Hepatic Disorders

Editor

Prof. Dr. P. H. Kulkarni

Sri Satguru Publications
A Division of
Indian Books Centre
Delhi, India

Published by
Sri Satguru Publications,
Indological and Oriental Publishers
A Division of
Indian Books Centre
40/5, Shakti Nagar,
Delhi-110007
India

Email: ibcindia@vsnl.com
Website: http://www.indianbookscentre.com

© Ayurveda Rasashala

First Edition; Pune 2001
Second Edition : Delhi 2001

ISBN 81-7030-720-1

Published by Sunil Gupta for Sri Satguru Publications, a division of Indian Books Centre, 40/5, Shakti Nagar, Delhi-110007, India and printed at Chawla Offset Printers, Delhi 110 052

A FEW WORDS OF GRATITUDE

During the Valedictory function of the last International Seminar, Prof. Dr.P.H. Kulkarni announced the theme and date of this seminar; at the same time to my great surprise he announced my name as an Organizing Secretary. Since then till this moment I was under tremendous pressure for the successful arrangement of the Seminar. But now I am the happiest person because the Seminar is about to conclude successfully.

I would like to mention my deepest gratitude towards none other than Prof. Dr.P.H. Kulkarni for the confidence he bestowed on in me. In addition I cannot describe in words the help and the guidance he gave in arranging this Seminar.

Any Seminar for its successful conclusion mostly depends on collected funds and delegation fees. For this very important task Dr.Suhas Parchure ably guided me and supported me wholeheartedly. I express my sincere thanks to him.

I want to express my special and sincere thanks to Dr.V.A.Dole (Vice Principal, Tilak Ayurveda Mahavidyalya). He has helped me in almost all the fields of work of the seminar. Whenever I approached him, he guided me without any hesitation. I never felt alone because I was confident that Dr. Dole was behind me.

While organizing various departments of this seminar I have to relinquish my duties at Tilak Ayurved Mahavidyalaya and Seth Tarachand Ramanath Hospital many times and I had to make necessary substitute arrangements. Dr V.V. Doiphode and Dr.B. K. Bhagwat, who were in charge of both these institutes during this period, kindheartedly permitted me to do so and gave me all the cooperation. I would like to be in their debt because I am sure they would not like mention of their names under official list of persons to be thanked.

To organize an International seminar on such a grand scale is not a job of a single person, it is teamwork and every member of the team must do his allotted work for the success of the seminar. I am very pleased to state that every member of the working committee has done his / her allotted job to my complete satisfaction and I have no hesitation to say that these persons have a lion's share in the success of the seminar. The members of the working committee are

Dr. Joglekar Vishnu
Dr. Pandhare Sunil
Dr. Pandit Sanjay
Dr. Mrs. Despande Manjiri
Dr. Mrs Patil Yogini
Dr. Gaikwad Manoj
Dr Mrs. Ujagare Indira
Dr. Mrs. Kadam Sujata
Dr. Barve Anand
Dr Patwardhan Manish
Dr. Mali Mahadeo
Dr. Miss Vanarse Monika
Dr. Miss Damale Anjali
Dr. Bhagwat Suvarna
Dr. Sarde Girish
Dr. Tillu Girish
Dr. Miss Tilay Darsha
Dr. Deshpande Sachin
Dr. Bhirud Nitin
Dr. Joglekar Priyadarshan

I am also thankful to,

Mr. Sagar Kulkarni, Mrs. Anuradha Wahegaonkar, Mrs. Yogini Kulkarni, Mr. Mahesh Gosawi, Mr. Godse (General Manager - Ayurveda RasaShala) and the whole team from Ayurveda Rasashala for their help.

Mr. Parag Joshi & Mr. Ashish Dudagikar for their pains taking efforts and neatness in Typography.

Mr. Ramesh Dhanokar of Green Graphics for printing and artwork.

Mr. Atul Nadagouda of Graphicon for printing and artwork. Milind Bhoi for efforts he has taken for publicity & propoganda of the seminar.

Teaching staff and Non-Teaching staff members of Tilak Ayurved Mahavidyalaya for their guidance and support.

Ayurved Rasashala and all the other Firms for their advertisements.

Dr.S.V.Deshpande

Jt.Organizer

Content

1	Hepatoprotective Effect Of Livocure In Acute Liver Damage - An Experimental Study. **Dr. Deshpande S. V.**	11
2	Abhyantara Vimargagamana Of Constituents With Respect To Yakruta & Its Management **Vaidya Ranjeet G. Nimbalkar**	21
3	Evaluation Of Hepatoprotective Actions Of Abhrak Bhasma In Albino Rats Against Hepatitis Induced By The Single Dose Of CCl4 **Savita Buwa**	27
4	Kumari Kalpa Ghansar Tablets Research With Microscopic High Resolution Blood Morphology Test (Peripheral Live Blood Analysis) In Chronic Fatigue Syndrome (CFS) **Dr. E.B.S. Premdani**	41
5	International Ayurveda Events	45
6	Liver Cancer Treatment As It Stands Today **Dr.Koppikar C.B.**	47
7	Chronic Hepatitis B Virus Infection **Dr Vinay K Thorat**	51
8	Clinical Interpretation Of LFT With Ayurvedic Point Of View. **Dr. Mali M. D.**	59
9	Introduction To Hepatitis 'C' And It's Ayurvedic Management **Vaidya Dhananjay J. Khajgiwale**	67
10	Hepatic Disorders And Imaging **Dr. Vilas A. Dole**	71
11	Clinical Evalution Of Phalatrikadi Kwath And Arogyavardhini In Early Hepatic Cirrhosis : A Case Report **Wachasundar Nachiket**	79
12	How To Treat Hepatitis With Ayurvedic Methods **Dr.Dandekar Govind**	83
13	Standerdisation Of Certain Ayurvedic Drugs Used For Kamala **A.Saraswathy**	87
14	Analysis Of Some Siddha Medicines Used For Kamala **A.Saraswathy**	88
15	Effect of Tamra Kumari In Liver Disorder **Vaidya Nikhil Kortikar**	89
16	Prevention of Liver Disease **Dr. Deepak Amarapurkar**	91
17	Liver Diseases & Homoeopathy **Dr. Hari Gholap**	93
18	Awareness Of Hepatotoxicity And Protectivity. **Dr. Lalitha B. R.**	97
19	Panchakarma Approach To Physio-pathological Problems Of Hepatitis (Yakritdalyodar) **Prof. Dr. T. Srinivas Rao**	101
20	Clinical Assessment Of Shankhabhasma Vati (Rasashala) + Laghusutshekhar Vati & Indrayav Vati In Amoebic Hepatitis **Vaidya P. C. Yawatkar**	105
21	Clinical Aspects Of Liver Disorders With Reference To Jalodar. **Vd. Ajit Joshi**	108

22	Copper Associated Childhood Cirrhosis **Dr. Avinash Pradhan**	112
23	Effect Of 'Stimuliv' In Viral Hepatitis **Dr. Mahesh Kagali**	114
24	Liver In Aquired Immune Deficiency Syndrome [AIDS] **Dr. Sanjay D. Deshmukh**	118
25	Treatment for Liver Disorders from Eye of Naturopathy **Dr.Sindhu Shiralkar**	120
26	Hepatitis Induced Ascites : A Clinical Study **Vd. Ashok G. Wali**	125
27	Role of Yakrit : Ayurvediya Vivechana. **Vd. Darsha Tilay**	131
28	Yakrddalyudara - Samprapti & Chikitsa **Dr.Monica Vanarase**	137
29	Liver Disorders and Their Ayurvedic Management **Vaidya Vilas Nanal**	142
30	Comparative Efficay Of Five Indigenous Compound Formulations In Patients Of Acute Viral Hepatitis. **S. V. Dange**	155
31	Effect Of Arogyavardhini – An Indigenous Compound Preparation, On Serum Lipids In Patients Of Acute Viral Hepatitis **S. V. Dange**	166
32	Role Of Liver In Skin Diseases **Dr. Milind Pendharkar**	173
33	A Proposed Hepato – Immuno Modulating Drug Regimen For Hepatitis. **Dr. M. V. Acharya**	176
34	Hepatic Disorders and Antioxidants: Mechanistic Aspects of Oxidative Injury and its Prevention by Garlic (Allium sativum, Linn.) unsaturated oils **Navneet Kumar Gupta**	178
35	Liver Dysfunction in Fetus : Hydrops Fetalis **Vd. P. C. Nagnoor**	191
36	Horoscope and Liver Disorders **Dr. Shrikant Bhide**	195
37	Hepatic Coma – Ayurvediya Management **Vd. M. D. Sane**	196
38	Roll Of Yakrita In Apasmara Chikitsa **Vd. V. S. Haldavnekar**	199
39	Herbal Applications In The Treatment Of Hepatic Aspects In Human Life **G. S. Chandras**	201
40	The Urgent For Hepatitis B Vaccination **Dr. S. Bhardwaj**	205
41	Vasadi Kashayam - My Drug of Choice in Kamala (Hepatitis) **Dr. Atulchandra Thombre**	206
42	Clinical Assessment Of Effect Of Kamalant In "Kamala" **Dr. Manohar J. Karachiwala**	208
43	Health Is A State Which We Create **Swami Joythirmayanand**	211
44	Importance Of Consideration Of Yakrut In The Treatment Of Sandhi Vikaras. **Vd. N. M. Pendse**	217
45	Alcoholic Hepatitis **Dr. Shobhana J. Bhatia**	218
46	Various Management of Rudhapath Kamala (Obstructive Jaundice) **Vd. Anant Dharmadhikari**	225
47	A Clinical Evaluation of an Ayurvedic Herbomineral Therapy in the Management of 120 Cases of Viral Hepatitis **Aashish S. Phadke**	228

*Hepatic Disorders*

Hepatoprotective Effect Of Livocure In Acute Liver Damage - An Experimental Study.

Dr. Mardikar B. R.
Dr. Deshpande S. V.

Abstract

Hepatoprotective effect of LIVOCURE was assessed against two chemical substances (Carbon tetrachloride, Paracetamol) which are known to cause hepatic damage and whose mechanism of action is also known to some extent. LIVOCURE effectively reversed the biochemical and histopathological changes in the liver induced by both hepatotoxins. In addition to its curative / corrective property, LIVOCURE also exerted a protective action enabling the hepatocytes to counteract the adverse effects of hepatotoxins.

Introduction

The liver plays a vital role in the metabolism and elimination of various endogenous and exogenous compounds. These biotransformation and detoxification processes expose the liver to various hepatotoxic agents.

Infections, drugs, alcohol and other dietary and environmental toxins induce structural and functional damage and predispose the liver to a vast array of disorders.

In the modern system of medicine there is no selective treatment of value for the management of hepato biliary disorders. In the absence of a universally acceptable and effective therapy, the management of hepato biliary disorders consists of supportive therapy in the form of bed rest, which provide only symptomatic relief to the patient and in most cases has no influence on the disease process.

Natural products, either singles or in combinations are proving successful day by day and it is almost agreed that the best line of treatment is with the various plant drug combinations.

LIVOCURE, is a herbal formulation (table 1 for composition) incorporating standardized extracts of proven hepato-protective of natural (herbal) origin, having antiinflammatory, choleretic, antifibrotic, immuno-modulatory and anti-viral actions, complimentary to its hepatoprotective effects.

Table 1

LIVOCURE TABLETS COMPOSITION

Each tablet contains extracts derived from:

Andrographis paniculata	250 mg
Picrorrhiza kurroa	250 mg
Phyllanthus niruri	300 mg
Boerhaavia diffusa	250 mg
Eclipta alba	250 mg
Tinospora cordifolia	250 mg
Glycyrrhiza glabra	250 mg

Materials & methods

Albino rats of weight range 80-110g body weight were used for the present study.

Rats were poisoned with Carbon tetrachloride and Paracetamol (sigma labs, Bombay) by intraperitoneal administration in the dose of 2ml / kg and 200 mg/kg respectively. A suspension prepared from LIVOCURE tablets supplied by Phyto medica, Bombay was administered in dose of 10gm/kg, by oral route. Carbon tetrachloride was mixed in refined Peanut oil (50 : 50).

The assessment of the efficacy was carried out with the help of biochemical estimation of various enzymes followed by histopathological observations. The results of the study are reported here.

Results

Hexabarbital sleeping time :

The normal sleeping time induced by hexabarbital was prolonged significantly by Carbon tetrachloride and Paracetamol administration. This was markedly shortened by the administration of LIVOCURE (**Fig.1**)

Serum Enzyme Studies

The rise in serum concentration of Alkaline phosphatase ($ALKPO_4$) and transaminases (SGOT, SGPT) was much lower in LIVOCURE – treated animals, than those receiving

Hepatic Disorders

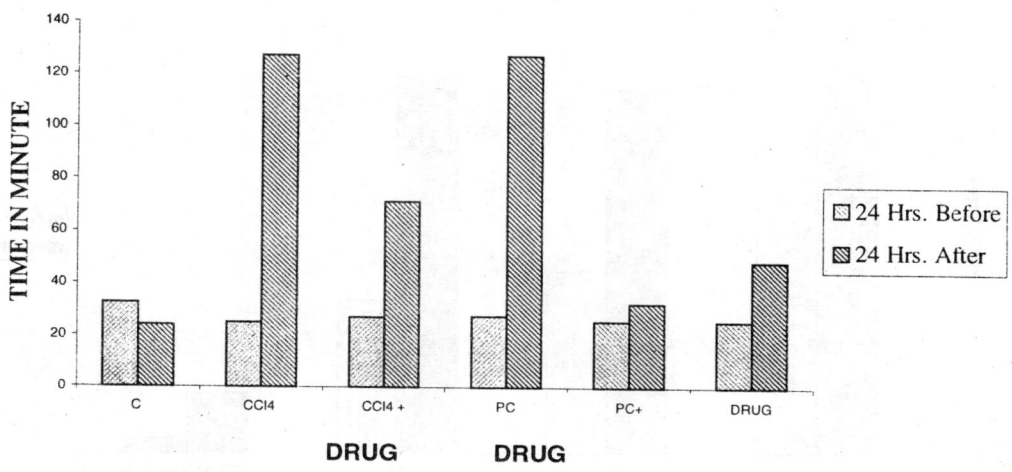

Bar Diagram Showing Hexabarbital Sleeping Time

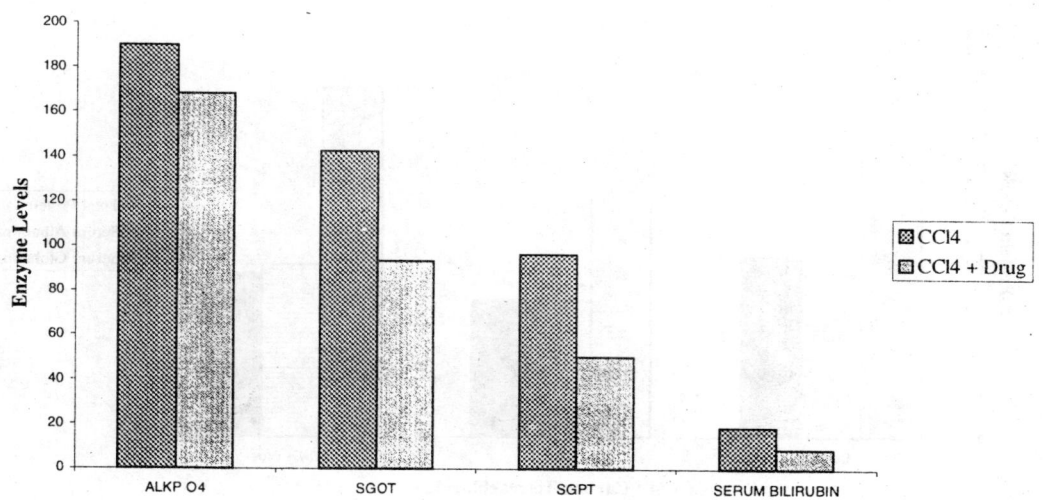

Bar Diagram Showing Enzymology in CCl4 & CCl4+ Drug Treated Groups

Hepatic Disorders

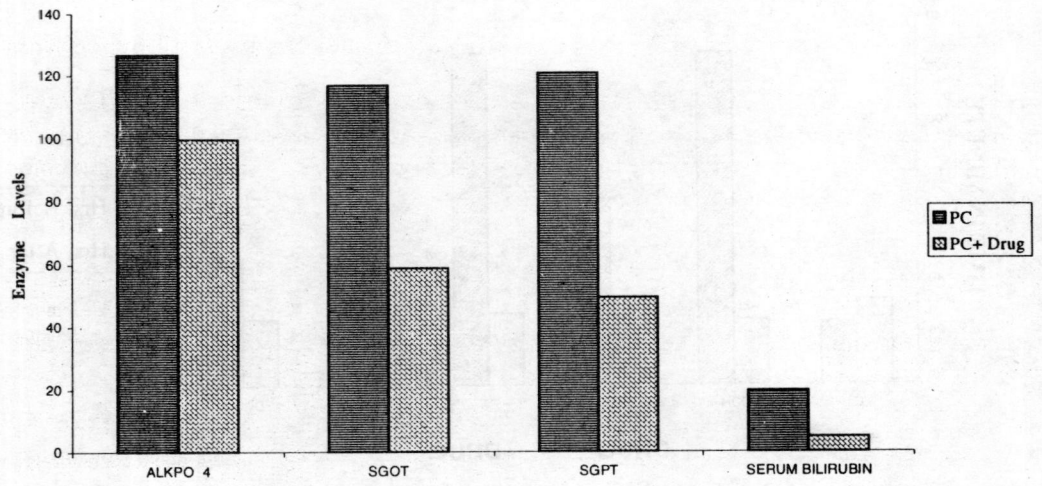

Bar Diagram Showing Enzymology In Paracetamol(PC), PC + Drug Treated Groups

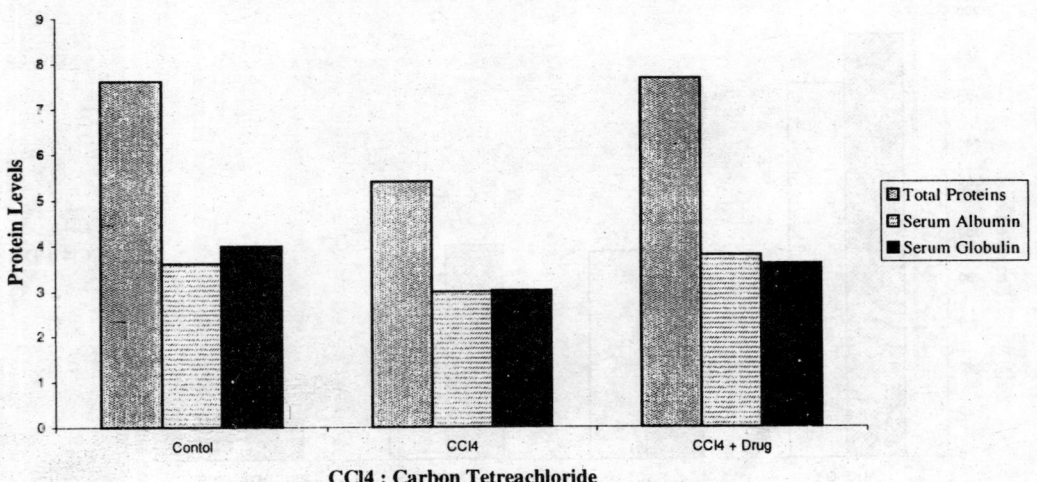

Bar Diagram Showing Protein Levels in CCl4 & CCl4 Drug Treated Groups

CCl4 : Carbon Tetreachloride

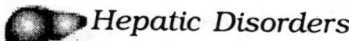
Hepatic Disorders

Bar Diagram Showing Protein Levels in Paracetamol (PC) & PC + Drug Treated Groups

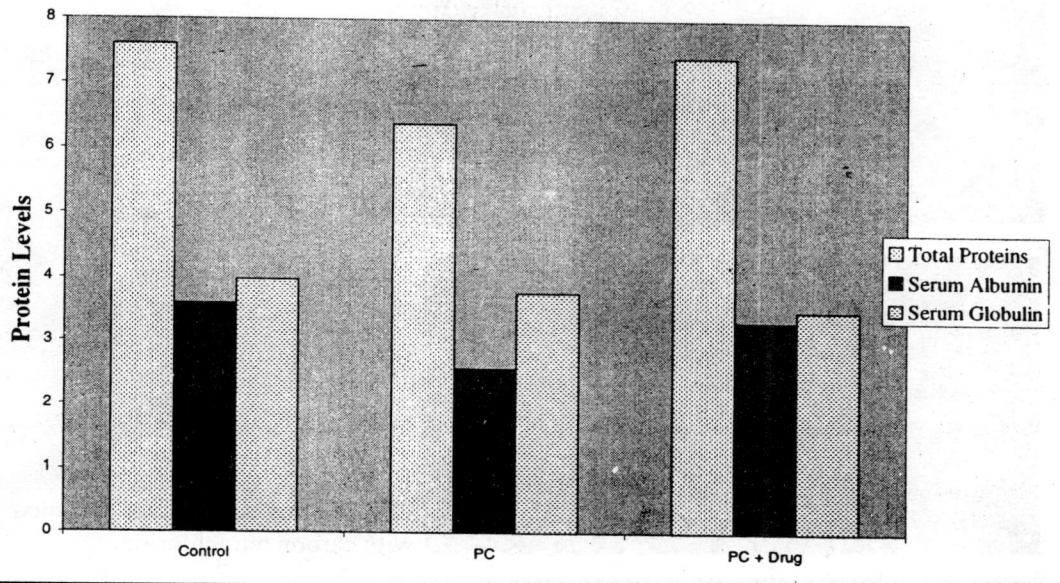

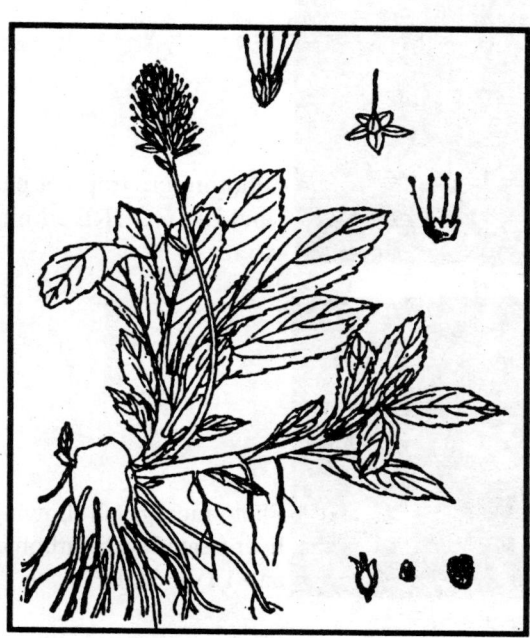

Sanskrit Name : Katuka
Latin Name : Picrorrhiza

Hepatic Disorders

Acute paracetamol damage

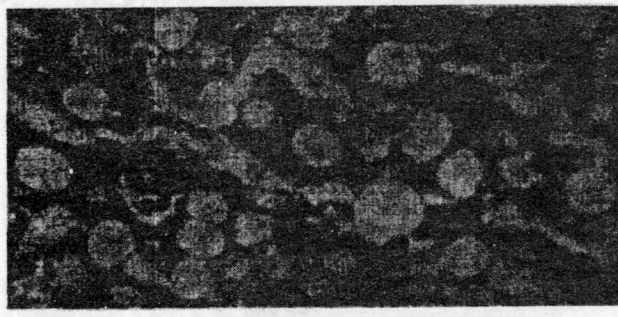

Photomicrograph of liver poisoned with carbon tetrachloride

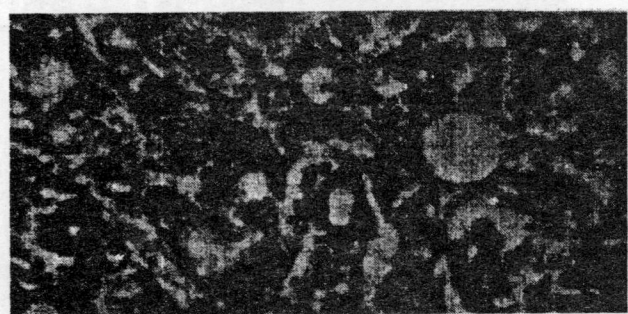

Photomicrograph of paracetamol and LIVOCURE administration to rat

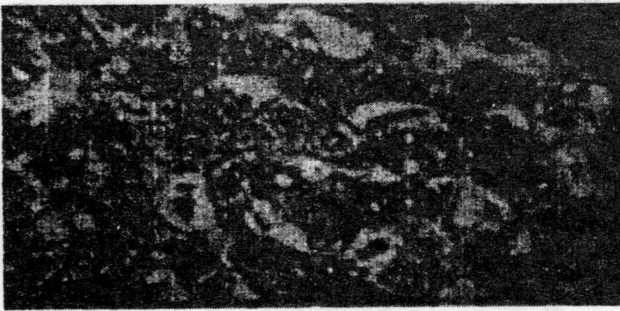

Photomicrograph showing the rat liver treated with carbontetrachloride and LIVOCURE

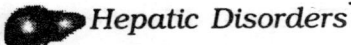*Hepatic Disorders*

Carbon tetrachloride and Paracetamol only (figs. 2 & 3).

Total Protein levels

There was a marked reduction in the Total protein, Albumin and Globulin levels in paracetamol and carbon tetrachloride treated animals. These levels returned to normal in LIVOCURE treated animals (figs 4 & 5).

Microscopic appearance

Histopathological sections of livers in paracetamol and carbon tetrachloride (figs. 6 & 7) treated groups showed damaged liver parenchyma, with centrilobular necrosis and fatty changes. The hepatocytes appeared smaller than normal with wider sinusoids and granular protoplasm.

Histopathological sections of livers in groups, treated with LIVOCURE, after inducing liver damage with hepatotoxins showed regeneration of hepatocytes, with complete disappearance of centrilobular necrosis, protoplasm being uniform with well spaced normal sinusoids. (figs. 8 & 9).

Discussion

In the present study, efficacy of LIVOCURE (Phyto medica) was tested against two chemical substances, which are known to cause hepatic damage, and whose mechanism of action is also known to some extent.

Carbon tetrachloride is an industrial toxin, which can cause massive hepatic damage in minute doses. The hepato-toxic effects of carbon tetrachloride depend upon the route of administration, amount employed and duration of treatment (Hartroft, 1964).

The acute changes in the liver produced by a single dose of carbon tetrachloride include centrilobular necrosis and fatty changes in parenchymal cells (Cameron and Karunaratne, 1936), while administration of small amounts over prolonged periods results in cirrhosis (Karandikar et al 1936; Mukherji and Wahi, 1968; Hase 1968; McLean et al 1969). Protection of liver against the acute toxic effects of Carbon tetrachloride has been shown using indigenous drugs and plants (Joglekar et al 1963; Srinivasan et al, 1968; Pandey and Chaturvedi, 1969).

Hence it can speculated that any drug which reverses the hepatic damage induced by Carbon tetrachloride can certainly protect liver parenchyma against other hepatotoxins. Paracetamol, a commonly used anti-pyretic, analgesic which is safe at therapeutic dose is reported to induce liver injury when used in large doses.

Thus, liver damage was produced in male albino rats with the help of Carbon tetrachloride by both oral and intraperitoneal route and the drug was administered simultaneously by oral route with the help of a metal cannula by the force feeding technique (photo page)

It is evident from the results that the differences in the values of control groups, challenge and challenge plus test drug are significantly different when student's 't' test is applied.

Carbon tetrachloride is known to cause liver damage by free radical formation during its metabolism by hepatic microsomes, which in turn cause peroxidation of cellular membranes leading to necrosis of hepatocytes & fatty liver. Since Carbon tetrachloride brings about hepatic damage by its action on the cell membrane and rough endoplasmic reticulum of the liver cells, it is tempting to speculate that LIVOCURE provides protective action by stabilizing the liver cell membrane or by protecting rough endoplasmic reticulum thereby decreasing lipid peroxidation and inhibiting microsomal enzymes.

Paracetamol produces liver injury through cholestatic effect. Paracetamol is mainly metabolized by glucuronide and sulphate conjugation. A small amount is metabolized by the cytochrome p450 system to a toxic metabolite. The cell is usually protected from injury by conjugation of this toxic metabolite with glutathione. As the dose increases, the glutathione content of the hepatocyte available for detoxification is exhausted and the hepatocyte becomes vulnerable to the noxious effects of the metabolite, resulting in liver cell necrosis.

LIVOCURE exerts hepatoprotective activity, probably by virtue of its ability to reduce lipoperoxides and increase Cytochrome P450 in the liver.

Estimation of transaminases is regarded as the most satisfactory method devised for determining hepatic function. It is one of the most sensitive and reliable among laboratory procedures for detecting minimal and early impairment of the function of the liver parenchyma. The rise in the activity of these enzymes reflects the degree of hepatocellular damage (Cantarow and Trumper, 1965; Sinha and Saran, 1972), leakage of large quantities of enzymes in to the blood stream being associated with massive necrosis of the liver (Rees and Spector, 1961).

The active regression of the raised transaminase values in the treated groups indicated the possibility of rapid liver cell regeneration by LIVOCURE against damage produced in the liver. Serum alkaline phosphatase, which is also a good indicator of hepatic function, also showed a marked increase in the unprotected group. This supported the view of active liver cell proliferation and commencing recovery of damaged liver cell proliferation and commencing recovery of damaged liver cells by LIVOCURE. The period of "Sleeping time" induced by short acting barbiturates is significantly prolonged in the event of any hepatic damage and this can be used as a measure of the function of the liver drug metabolizing enzymes. Our results infer that significantly shorten hexabarbital "Sleeping time" as compared to animals receiving Carbon tetrachloride & paracetamol respectively, thus confirming its protection of hepatic drug metabolizing enzymes.

These effects of LIVOCURE cannot be attributed to any single chemical compound.

Hepatic Disorders

Obviously it is due to the synergistic action of multiple active principles contained in the various herbal ingredients.

Conclusion

The present animal experiments do tell us very vividly that LIVOCURE certainly offers a protective action to the hepatocytes, which have the ability to reverse the toxic effects of Carbon tetrachloride and Paracetamol on mammalian liver cells.

In our opinion, LIVOCURE is a highly promising Ayurvedic herbal combination, which can be used, in various acute and chronic liver diseases.

Acknowledgements

We are grateful to Mr. Kishor Shah, Director, M/s. Phyto medica, Bombay for encouraging this study. We also thank the medical advisor of this company, Dr. V. V. R. Durga Prasad. We thank the laboratory staff of our institution for very prompt analytical work.

Bibliography

1. Charak Samhita
2. Sushrut Samhita
3. Ashtanga Sangraha
4. Nadkarni, Indian Materia Medica, Vol I
5. Bhavaprakash
6. Nighantu Ratnakar
7. Kaiyya Dev Nighantu
8. Chikitsa Pradeep
9. Kirtikar & Basu, B.D.
10. Hartroft, 1964
11. Cameron & Karunaratne, 1936
12. Karandikar et al, 1936
13. Mukherji & Wahi, 1968
14. Hase, 1968
15. Mclean et al, 1969
16. Joglekar et al, 1963
17. Srinivasan et al, 1968
18. Pandey & Chaturvedi, 1969
19. Cantarow & Trumper, 1965

Hepatic Disorders

20. Sinha & Saran, 1972
21. Rees & Spector, 1961
22. Mahrotra R. et al. Ind.J.Med. Res. 92(B), (1990), 133
23. Thyagarajan, S.P. et al Ind.J.Med. Res. 76((Suppl.), (1982), 124.
24. Venkateshwaran P. S. et al Proc.Nat.Acad.Sc. Washington 84(1), (1987). 274
25. Thyagarajan, S.P. et al; The Lancet, (1988), 864
26. Pandey V. N. et al Ind. J. Med. Res. 57(3), (1969), 503
27. Das P. K. et al, Ind. J. Exp. Biol. 14(4), (1976), 456
28. Dwivedi Y. et al. Ind. J. Med. Res. 92 (B), (1990), 195
29. Handa S.S et al Ind. J. Med. Res. 92 (B), (1990), 236
30. Handa, S. S. et al Fitoterapia 57(5), (1986), 336

Dr. Mardikar B. R.
Ex-Principal, College of Ayurved, Bharati Vidyapeeth, Erandawane, Pune 411 038.
Dr. Deshpande S. V.
B.A.M.S., M.D., Ph.D.(AYUR.) H.O.D. Kayachikitsa, Tilak Ayurved Mahavidyalaya, Pune 411011.

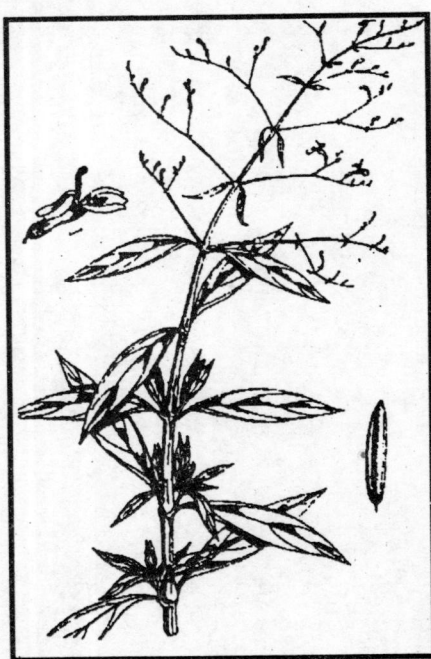

Sanskrit Name : Kalamegh
Latin Name : Andrographis paniculata

Hepatic Disorders

Abhyantara Vimargagamana Of Constituents With Respect To Yakruta & Its Management

Vaidya Ranjeet G. Nimbalkar

In the body, the basic constituents are doshas, dhatus & malas. Each of them is flowing in its respective pathway & carrying out its physiological functions. These pathways are called as srotasas.

Because of some causes, the srotasas are vitiated & cannot perform their normal functions. This vitiation shows 4 types of symptoms, as follows:-

अतिप्रवृत्तिः संगो वा शिराणां ग्रन्थयोऽपि वा ।

विमार्गगमनं चापि स्रोतसां दुष्टिलक्षणम् ॥ च.वि. ९

I.e.
- (i) Overflow of the constituents of the srotasa
- (ii) Reduced flow of the constituents
- (iii) Blockage of channels due to clots (granthi)
- (iv) Change of path (vimargagamana) of constituents.

Now, as we know, vimargagamana is abnormal flow of constituents in other srotasas, resulting in abnormal accumulation of that constituent in the srotas in which it is abnormally flowing. Also it causes its deficiency in its own srotasa.

We see in detail, its types, effects on the physiology & its importance in deciding the line of treatment of that particular disease.

The Vimargagamana can be considered of 2 types

viz.
- (I) Mechanical & Non-mechanical
- (II) Bahya & Abhyantara

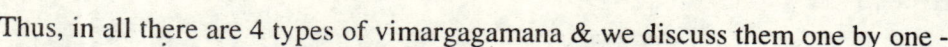
Hepatic Disorders

Thus, in all there are 4 types of vimargagamana & we discuss them one by one -

(i) **Mechanical & bahya vimargagamana** - In this case there is mechanical or anatomical deformity in the srotas & because of that the constituents, not belonging to that srotasa, flow in it & are **visible** in the clinical examination.

The commonest example is the vesico-vaginal fistula, where, there is formation of a direct pathway between urethra & vagina of the female. As a result, passage of urine is through vaginal orfice.

(ii) **Mechanical & Abhyantara vimargagamana** - In this case also, there is anatomical defect in the srotasas, causing abnormal flow of constituents, which is not visible directly. In the clinical assessment. We have to use special techniques to find it, or rely on symptoms.

The commonest examples are various congenital anomalies of the heart e.g. ASD, VSD, PDA etc.

The above two types are mainly the subjects of surgery & surgical procedures maybe needed for their correction.

(iii) **Non-mechanical & bahya vimargagamana** - In this case, there is no anatomical deformity in the srotasas, but still, due to physiological defect, constituents change their path & are **seen** flowing in other srotasa.

The commonest example is Atisara, where Udaka dhatu from udakawaha srotasa is misdirected in the purishavaha srotasa & excreted.

(iv) **Non-mechanical & abhyantara vimargagamana** - Here, of course, there is no mechanical deformity & also no visible evidence of vimargagamana. We have to locate such phenomenon by keen observations & yukti pramana.

The last 2 cases are the subjects of kaya chikitsa & the last i.e. non-mechanical & abhyantara vimargagamana is the topic of this paper.

There is no specific term used as abhyantara vimargagamana in the texts, but as we read the texts, between the lines, we get a clear-cut concept, about this phenomenon, & we can implement it in treating various other diseases, which are not responding to conventional treatment.

As the subject is limited for Yakruta only. First we study the diseases, showing vimargagamana phenomena & are related to yakrita. Three such main diseases, which show seeds of this phenomena are - Kamala, Raktapita & Yakrutodara.

(i) **Kamala** - In any type of kamala, depending upon the cause (Bahupitta or

Hepatic Disorders

Margavarodhaja), there is vimargagamana of Raktamala pitta into Raktavaha srotasa. i.e. Pitta, which should be going to Annavaha srotasa & excreted through Purishavaha srotasa, due to some abnormality of yakruta, flows into the rakta & then to all the body.

(ii) **Raktapitta** - In case of Raktapitta, liquid part of various dhatus, because of excessive heat of pitta, drains into Rakta, increasing its quantity. This is vimargagamana of Uadaka of various dhatus in Rakta, because of some functional abnormality of yakruta.

तस्योष्मणा द्रवो धातुर्धातोर्धातो: प्रसिच्यते ।

स्विद्यतस्तेन संवृद्धि भूयस्तदधिगच्छति ॥ च.चि. ४/८

(iii) **Yakrutodara** - The samprapti of Yakrutodara & pleehodara is the same, which tells that -

वामपार्श्वाश्रित: प्लीहा च्युत: स्थानाद्विवर्धते ।

शोणितं वा रसादिभ्यो विवृद्धं तं विवर्धयेत् ॥ वा.नि. १२/२४

The enlargement of liver is due to increased quantity of Rakta. The causes of quantitative increase in Rakta are the drainage of udaka from other dhatus (शोणितं वा रसादिभ्य:) in Rakta.

Thus, it is clear that the internal disturbances in the flow of various constituents, resulting in their vimargagamana are common, and roots of that particular srotasas are the cause for it & the srotasa in which the vimargaga constituents are coming, is also affected.

Rasa & Rakta, being liquid dhatus are more prone for vimargagamana. Also Rasa & Rakta dhatus are responsible for nourishment of all the other dhatus. This is also the cause, because if the nourishment (i.e. poshaka dhatu) is not accepted by the poshya dhatu, its vimargagamana takes place, resulting in its accumulation in Rasa or Raktavaha srotas & malnourishment of that particular dhatu.

After studying this conceptual discussion, we study a pathological condition in which liver involvement is common, & we have to think of vimargagamana of dhatus, with respect to liver. This is Fatty degeneration of liver, due to alcohol.

(i) **Fatty degeneration of liver** - We first see the pathology described by the modern medicine. Under controlled conditions, alcohol administration has been shown to produce hepatic fatty change, regularly in man. After a single dose of alcohol, the fatty acids, which accumulate in the liver are derived from fat depos, whereas in chronic alcohol intake, they are predominantly of dietary origin.

Alcohol is broken down by oxidation & generation of Hydrogen ions, causing resultant

Hepatic Disorders

change in reduction & oxidation (Redox) potential. Also there is proliferation of smooth endoplasmic reticulum & is a well recognized feature of alcoholic liver damage & it seems that induction of a no of microsomal enzyme systems may accompany this increase & contribute to some of the other effects of alcohol on hepatocyte fat metabolize. In addition, motochandria are damaged by alcohol, they become swolle, producing giant forms.

Because of these changes, there is accumulation of fatty acids in the hepatocytes, due to altered redox potential. This is aggravated by direct damage to mitochondria. Also increased a - glycerophosphatase results in trapping of fatty acids in the hepatocytes. These fatty acids are then esterified in endoplasmic reticulum to triglycerides.

Cholesterol esters also accumulate & is partly due to increased cholesterol production & partly due to reduced, cholesterol catabolism.

These mechanisms combine to produce fatty change, demonstrable even after 2 days of alcohol consumption. Stopping alcohol results in rapid mobilization of fat from hepatocytes. But chronic alcohol consumption leads to the permanent liver changes.

Ayurveda explains this fat deposition in an altogether different way.

According to Ayurveda, liver or yakruta, is an organ made from Rakta in the fetal life.

गर्भस्य यकृत्प्लीहानौ शोणितजौ । सु.शा. ४

Also Yakruta is a moola of Rakta vaha srotasa. This any vikruti or pathology of yakruta affects Rakta & vice versa.

Madya is considered as a visha of low power

तीक्ष्णादयो विषेऽप्युक्ताश्चित्तोपप्लाविनो गुणाः ।
जीवितान्ताय जायन्ते विषे तूत्कर्ष वृत्तितः ॥ वा.नि.

Thus Madya, being a visha, when taken regularly, even in small amounts, is bound to vitiate all the dhatus, especially Rakta.

तीक्ष्णोष्णरूक्षसूक्ष्माम्लं व्यवाय्याशुकरो लघुः ।
विकाशि विशदं मद्यमोजसोऽस्मादद्विपर्ययः ॥ वा.नि.

All the gunas of Madya are capable of vitiation of Rakta.

The excess of Tikshana, Ushna, Rooksha, Sookshma, Amla, Vyavayi, laghu etc. gunas, produce Vidaha of Rakta. i.e. production of excess of Tikshana & Ushna gunas in Rakta. Also these gunas cause vitiation of Pitta & Vata.

Hepatic Disorders

Because of vitiation of Vata, Pitta & Rakta & excess of heat in the body, Swedana of all the other dhatus is effected & these dhatus lose their drava part along with their poshaka anshas. All these are drained & accumulated in Rakta, as we have seen in Raktapitta & Yakrutodara samprapti.

Because of Laghu Khara gunas, along with Ushna & Tikshna, maximum nourishing parts (poshaka anshas) of Mamsa & Meda, are drained in the Rakta. When such Rakta is going into Yakruta for processing, the disabled yakruta cannot get rid of these dhatus & they start accumulating in the khavaigunya of the yakruta (caused may be due to previous incidences or even due to excess alcohol).

Thus this is a classical example of vimargagama of Mamsa & Meda dhatus into Raktavaha srotasa. Excess of these dhatus, especially meda in yakruta, slowly result in its enlargement.

Also due to vimargagamana of poshaka parts of Mamsa & Meda into Yakruta, the poshya or sthayi dhatus do not get their nourishment & there is gradual reduction in their quantity & quality. This fact explains the cachexic appearance of the chronic alcoholic patient.

When we come to the treatment part, importance of the above samprapti can be understood. If we use Rooksha & Laghu dravyas for Lekhana of Meda, accumulated in Yakruta, it will be a great mistake, because due to such medicines, the condition of the patient will be worsened.

So while treating such patients, initially the treatment should be brinhana, because -

बृंहणं शमनं त्वेव वायोः पित्तानिलस्य च । वा.सू. ९४

But if the brinhana treatment is given blindly, then also the condition will be worsened because more & more fat accumulation will take place in the liver & cachexia of the patient will be persistent. Therefore to correct the vimargagamana, should be the first & the foremost stage. The chief dosha of any normal or abnormal movement in the body is vata dosha. Thus to correct vimargagamana, the first step should be correction of vata.

The best known method for correction of vitiated vata is basti. Along with Anuvasana & Niruha bastis, proper use of brinhana bastis can be done. Brinhana bastis should only be used after correction of gati of Vata. This correction can be easily understood by regularization of appetite & bowel habits, sleep, pain reduction & increase in the activities (Utsaha) of the patient.

The medicines chosen for brinhan basti should be such that -

(i) They should not cause overfilling (Sampoorana)
(ii) They should also act on Rakta.

The best medicines completing the above criteria are Ananta, Yastimadhu & Bala. They

Hepatic Disorders

are sheeta & not ushna like Ashwagandha & Kapikacchu & they are not over nourishing like Shatavari.

Thus proper use of these medicines, prepared in milk & ghee for brinhan basti will also reduce the vidaha of Rakta & Pitta. As this vidaha reduces, automatically swedana of dhatus will be reduced & further drain of dhatus is stopped.

Lastly, for the meda, which is originally accumulated, Laghu, Ushna, Khara (i.e. Lekhana) type of medicines can be used, along with the above treatment & continuous assessment of tolerance of the patient to the treatment.

Thus the line of treatment for any vimargagamana will be -

(i) Correction of vata
(ii) Correction of Khavaigunya, of the srotasa, in which vimargagamana has taken place.
(iii) Correction of vimargagata bhava padartha.

Vaidya Nimbalkar Ranjit Ganpat
721/2B, Vikas Nagar, Navi Peth, Pune – 411 030 Tel. : 4336130

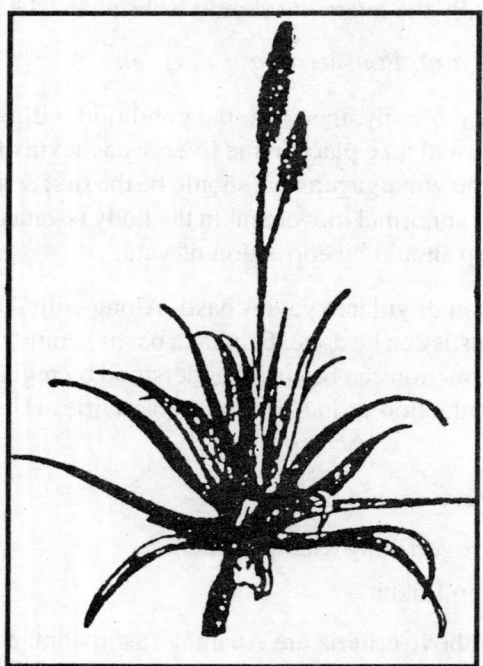

Sanskrit Name : Kumari
Latin Name : Aloe vera

*Hepatic Disorders*

Evaluation Of Hepatoprotective Actions Of Abhrak Bhasma In Albino Rats Against Hepatitis Induced By The Single Dose Of CCl_4

Savita Buwa, P. H. Kulkarni.
Aruna Kanase, Subhash Patil.

Abhrak Bhasma is a commonly used Ayurvedic drug against many diseases including hepatitis. It is tested in albino rats using a model of hepatitis induced by a single dose of CCI4 [3 ml/Kg body weight]. Different doses of Abhrak bhasma [10, 20, 30 and 40 mg/Kg body Wt] were tested to decide the dose related hepatoprotective efficacy. The centrilobular necrosis induced by single dose of CCl_4 was reduced significantly by 10 mg Abhrak bhasma and liver histology was almost protected by 20 mg dose. Liver acid lipase activity was lowered, while alkaline and lipoprotein lipase activities were elevated due to treatment of single dose of CCl_4. Abhrak bhasma counteracted the action of CCl_4 liver lipolytic enzymes. CCl_4 did not alter the Kidney histologically. The activities of all three lipases of rat kidney, acid, alkaline and lipoprotein lipases were reduced by CCl_4 treatment. The action of CCl_4 on kidney lipases was reversed by the administration of Abhrak bhasma. Acid lipase activity of rat adipose tissue was reduced by CCl_4 treatment. On the contrary alkaline, lipoprotein and hormone sensitive lipases were enhanced 24 hours after the administration of CCl_4 Acid lipase activity was raised by the administration of different dose of Abhrak bhasma concurrent with CCl_4. Abhrak bhasma treatment along with CCl_4 enhanced alkaline lipase activity at 10 and 20 mg dose and later it was reduced at 30 and 40 mg doses and brought towards normal level. Lipoprotein and hormone sensitive lipases were reduced by the counteraction of increasing doses of Abhrak bhasma. The possible significance of lipases I Abhrak bhasma mediated hepatoprotection is discussed.

Lipases play roles in lipid metabolism and lipid turnover. Lipoprotein lipase [LPL] degrades chylomicrons and free fatty acids are uptaken by the different tissues[1,2]. Hormone sensitive lipase [HSL] hydrolyzes triglycerides to monoglycerides for their mobilization from adipose tissue to different tissues and cells[3-5]. Hepatic lysosomal lipase/acid lipase [ACL][6-10] is involved in the degradation of lipid material for recirculation of fatty acids. Alkaline lipase is supposed to be microsomal and cytosolic[8,9,11,12] and is involved in lipid synthesis. Our earlier work on lipolytic activities during hepatoprotection mediated by different ayurvedic drugs has shown that the lipases are influenced by the status of hepatitis, hepatoprotection by ayurvedic drugs and corresponding altered physiology of the animals. Mandur bhasma [10 mg/kg body wt; PO] administration to CCl_4 + liquid paraffin [CCl_4 in liquid paraffin 3:1 v/v/kg body wt.] treated rats for 11 days resulted in hepatoprotection through regeneration of liver evidence by mitosis coupled with renal protection too[13]. Liver lipoprotein lipase was increased enhancing the secretion hepatic of lipoproteins coupled with lowered acid lipase and hormone sensitive lipase [to indicate less lipolysis than uptake of fatty acids]. CCl_4 induced lowered activities of lysosomal acid lipases from liver and kidney counteracted by mandur bhasma by releasing fatty acids for regeneration with increased activities of alkaline lipases which are also needed for regeneration. Patil *et. al*[14] showed similar alterations in activities of acid, lipoprotein and hormone sensitive lipases during Kumari asav, Kumari kalpa, Arogyavardhini and Tamra bhasma mediated differential hepatoprotection when these drugs were given to the rats simultaneous with CCl_4 for 7 days. These four ayurvedic drugs when used in the other mode of toxicity where CCl_4 was administered once in a week for 4 weeks [15] the alkaline lipase activity was decreased but, lipoprotein lipase and hormone sensitive lipase activities were increased. These differences in the alterations were attributed to the modes of toxicities. Single dose of CCl_4 induces acute centrilobular necrosis[16] and alters the lipid metabolism. CCl_4 [0.1 ml/100gm body wt.] introduced intraduodenally increased liver tri-and di-glycerides levels after 24 hrs in albino rats with centrilobular necrosis, which were influenced by dietary lipids[17]. But 0.5ml CCl_4/100 g body wt also elevated the levels of medium c-chain fatty acids [which were decreased by lipid balanced diet] in adipose tissue and not in liver and decreased saturated fatty acids [without any alteration in dietary linoleic acid and linolenic acid] in rat. The repair mechanisms are influenced by phospholipids [phosphotidylcholine being more pronounced in action][18] and coupled with rise in levels of thymidylate synthetase and thymidine kinase in liver with reaching at peaks at 72 hrs indicating liver regeneration[19]. Thus lipid metabolism is influenced by both toxicity by CCl_4 and regeneration of liver.

Material and methods

Abhrak bhasma was prepared in the laboratory as described earlier in material and methods. Albino rats were bred and reared in departmental animal house. The rats were originally derived from Haffkine stain. They were provided Standard pellet feed [Amrit rat feed prepared by Navbharat Chakan Oil Mills, Sangli, India] and water *ad libitum*. The rats weighing 130 to 140 g were used for the present experiment. The animals were grouped into 6 groups [each containing 8 animals]. The rats of first group were designated as normal and were not given any treatment. The rats of the groups 2 to 6 were given injections of CCl_4 between 8-00 to 9-00 a.m. only once. The rats of the groups 3 to 6 were given orally 10, 20, 30 and 40 mg/kg body wt Abhrak bhasma respectively, immediately after the injection of CCl_4. Later food was supplied to the animals. They were deprived of food 1 hrs prior to killing. The rats were killed after 24 hrs by giving deep ether anesthesia. The livers, kidneys and adipose tissues were dissected out. The pieces of livers and kidneys were fixed in fixative containing 4% paraformaldehyde and 1% glutaraldehyde in 0.2 M phosphate buffer at pH 7.00, processed for the preparation of paraffin blocks, the sections were cut at 5m and stained with hematoxylin and eosin and Mallory triple stain. The tissues were homogenized and diluted to a suitable volume with distilled water. And used for the assays of lipases. Acid lipase was determined according to the method of Mahadevan and Tappel[8] and alkaline, lipoprotein and hormone sensitive lipase were assayed in tissue homogenates as described earlier by Matsumura et al[21] using triolein as a substrate. The enzyme activities were terminated at the end of incubation period. The fatty acids liberated were estimated as described by Itaya[22]. The proteins of lives and kidneys were estimated using Folin phenol reagent[23]. Proteins from adipose tissues were estimated using the method described by Tornqvist and Belfrage[24]. Students t-test was carried out according to Agarwal[25].

Results and discussion

Single dose causes centrilobular necrosis in liver and figures depict alterations in the region. Periarterial region remained normal with the treatment of 3.0 ml/kg dose of CCl_4. Kidney histology was not altered by single dose. Normal arrangement of cetrolobular lobule is well studied earlier[26]. The hepatic cells radially arranged in hepatic cords. Sinusoids perforated the hepatic cords and sinusoidal and Kupffer cells were distributed through the lobule (fig. 1). Bile canaliculi were clear. Hepatocytes were distinct due to their large shape and staining. Nuclei were basophilic and placed in central region of cells. Cytoplasm is eosinophilic. This arrangement was altered by CCl_4 treatment (fig.2). Single dose of CCl_4 induced necrosis in hepatic cells and distorted the hepatic cords, blocked the variations from small spherical to large droplet like structures. In most of the necrotic cells the centrally placed nuclei were suspended in small amount of cytoplasm which remains continuous by cytoplasmic strands that traverse through the vacuoles connecting the peripheral rim of cytoplasm. Many of them were advancing towards death/dead. Kupffer cells and sinusoidal cells showed arrest in distribution. It was studied earlier and described as hydropic degeneration/fatty degeneration[16, 27, 28]. Ten mg Abhrak bhasma given orally simultaneous with CCl_4 protected the liver partially (fig. 3). The centrilobular region showed necrosis, but the extent of the area of necrotic region was reduced significantly. Numbers of necrotic cells located in this region were considerably reduced and were retained in immediate vicinity of the vein. Most of the cells on the boundary of the necrotic region show small vacuoles indicating preliminary stage of necrosis. The area of healthy cells and necrotic cells were located in the same lobular region. Necrotic region showed the pathological architecture as described above and in region of healthy cells normal histological structure was evident. In centrilobular region of CCl_4 + Abhrak bhasma [20 mg] treated rats the region was normal without any necrotic cells or the cells that show any type of stress (Fig. 4). Clear bile canaliculi were noted. Distribution of Kupffer cells and sinusoidal cells was normal. The liver was totally normal by the treatments of 30 and 40 mg Abhrak bhasma/kg body wt

Hepatic Disorders

concomitant with CCl_4. The histological alterations have clearly indicated that 20 mg of Abhrak bhasma protects the CCl_4 induced centrilobular necrosis. Similar type of hepatoprotection against CCl_4 was also noted by Tamra bhasma[29].

Rise in liver weight and fall in adipose tissue wt occurred 24 hrs after single injection of CCl_4, but kidney wt did not altered (Table 1). Increasing doses of Abhrak bhasma counteracted the action of CCl_4 by reducing the liver wt. The wet of the kidney was reduced in group 3 to 6 when compared to that of group 1 and 2 rats. It was lowest in group 4 rats. Treatment of Abhrak bhasma to CCl_4 treated rats further reduced the wet wt of the adipose tissues of group 3 and 4 rats, then it was raised in group 5 and 6 rats. The wt of group 6 rat adipose tissue was significantly higher than that of normal and CCl_4 treated rat. Group 6 rats exhibited the highest wt of adipose tissue as compared to the values observed in the rats other groups.

Acid and alkaline lipases of rat liver were declined by the treatment of CCl_4, however conspicuous rise in lipoprotein lipase activity was noted (Table 2). Administration of Abhrak bhasma along with CCl_4 resulted in rise in acid and lipoprotein lipase activities in group 3 to 6 rats when compared to the corresponding values of group 2 rat liver, except acid lipase activity of group 6 rat liver. Lipoprotein lipase activities were markedly greater than normal values. Similarly acid lipase activities of group 5 rat liver were higher than the normal values. The administration of 10 mg/kg body wt Abhrak bhasma concomitant with CCl_4 to group 3 rats enhanced lipoprotein lipase activity. as compared to the normal value and that of only CCl_4 treated rats. Alkaline lipase was lower in group 4 and 5 rat liver than the values observed in normal and CCl_4 treated rats. Alkaline lipase activity of group 6 rat liver was nearer to the normal value.

Administration of single dose of CCl_4 reduced all the three lipases of rat kidneys (Table 3). The activities were low when expressed per g tissue as well as per mg protein. Increasing doses of Abhrak bhasma simultaneous with CCl_4 (given of the rats of groups 3 to 6) elevated acid lipase activities in response to the doses. Similar observations were noted in alkaline lipases of rat kidneys of the groups 3 to 6, excepting the enzyme activity per mg protein of group 5 rats, which was below the corresponding value observed in group 4 rat kidney. This may be due to marked rises in protein content of group 5 rat kidney. Lipoprotein lipase activities per g tissue were conspicuously low in group 2 rat kidneys than normal value. Abhrak bhasma counteracted the action of CCl_4 by enhancing the enzyme activity. When lipoprotein lipase activities of the rats of the groups 3, 4 and 5 were expressed as per mg protein exhibited the results parallel to the corresponding enzyme activity per g tissue. While lipoprotein lipase activity of group 5 rat kidney were lower than that noted in the kidneys of the rats of groups 1, 3, 4 and 5 and lower then the value seen in group 2 rat kidney.

Sharp rises in alkaline, lipoprotein and hormone sensitive lipases of adipose tissue were noted after the single injection of CCl_4 to the rats of group 2 along with significant fall in acid lipase activity (table 4). Administration of 10 mg/kg body wt Abhrak bhasma enhanced acid and alkaline lipases (after expressing both as per g tissue and per mg tissue) as compared to the corresponding values in group 2 rats. Acid and alkaline lipases were declined with increasing doses o Abhrak bhasma administered to the rats of groups 4 to 6. Parallel changes were noted after expressing the enzyme activities as either per g tissue or per mg protein. Treatments of ascending doses of Abhrak bhasma concomitant with CCl_4 reduced the activities of lipoprotein and hormone sensitive lipases per g tissue and per mg protein as compared to the respective values noted in group2 rat adipose tissue, excepting lipoprotein and hormone sensitive lipase activities per mg protein of group 3 and 5 rat adipose tissues respectively.

Carbon tetrachloride treatment causes accumulation of lipids in the liver and kidney[16]. It is suggested that lipids from peripheral adipose tissue are translocated to liver and kidney for accumulation[16]. It has been also shown in this laboratory that lipases play important role in hepatic necrosis[13-15]. As in our earlier work, acid and alkaline lipases of liver were reduced after the administration of single dose of CCl_4 during present study. Similar fall in acid lipase and accumulation of triacylglycerol were noted in rat hepatocytes in primary culture in the presence of CCl_4[30]. Reduction in alkaline lipase indicated the damage to ER since it is bound to ER[7,11,31,32] and CCl_4 damages smooth ER. Higher activity of liver lipoprotein lipase may indicate the increased secretion of lipoprotein and high turnover of lipoproteins as the later period after the administration of CCl_4. This increase may be attributed to the stimulation of tissue repair since at later periods (24 hrs) after CCl_4 injection, both the damage and recovery proceed simultaneously[33]. However it was inhibited by repeated doses of CCl_4[13]. Progressive histological recovery and enhanced acid lipase activity of liver by oral administration of increasing doses of Abhrak bhasma concomitant with CCl_4 indicate that degradation of accumulated lipids during hepatoprotection (which are translocated due to CCl_4 toxicity) lipids are hydrolyzed by lysosomal lipase at faster rate preventing lipid accumulation. Linear rise in acid lipase activity was notes in groups 3 to 5 and declined in group 6 rat liver. These results suggest that during progressive hepatoprotection acid lipase activity rises and in during total hepatoprotection it tends towards the normal value. Rise in alkaline lipase activity as a function of dose of Abhrak bhasma suggest the recovery of endoplasmic reticulum which was supported by histological recovery at 20 to 40 mg. Lipoprotein lipase activities exhibited the alterations parallel to alkaline lipase activities suggesting the improvement in lipoprotein metabolism.

All lipases of the kidney of group 2 rats were suppressed by CCl_4 treatment deteriorating lipid metabolism. Similar observations were noted earlier after the administration of CCl_4 in liquid paraffin for 11 days[13]. Administration of increasing doses of Abhrak bhasma raised all the lipases. Higher acid lipase activity suggests the increased degradation of cellular accumulated lipids. However rises in alkaline lipase activities and lipoprotein lipase activities after Abhrak bhasma treatment along with CCl_4 indicated the higher uptake and turnover of lipids to overcome the stress induced by CCl_4. This can be attributed to high energy turnover in kidney during hepatoprotection.

Acid lipase activity of adipose tissue was inhibited by the administration of CCl_4. While the activities alkaline, lipoprotein and hormone sensitive lipases were higher 24 hrs after the injection of CCl_4 suggests the mobilization of lipids from adipose tissue for accumulation during CCl_4 toxicity. Similar observations noted in our earlier work in this laboratory[13-15]. The present results indicate high turnover of lipids 24 hrs after CCl_4 injection. All lipases increased in group 3 and 4 rat adipose tissues and brought towards normal values (although they were higher than normal values) in groups 5 and 6 in response to higher doses of Abhrak bhasma. Partial hepatoprotection was noted in group 3 rat, all most all liver recovery was observed in group 4 rats and total hepatoprotection was seen in groups 5 and 6 rats. The alterations in wet weight and lipase activities suggest that during hepatoprotection turnover of lipids occur while as the liver recovery progresses the lipid turnover declines, although it was higher than normal. All the lipases exhibit similar behavior after the administration of increasing doses of Abhrak bhasma concurrent with CCl_4.

Abhrak bhasma is an amorphous powdery ayurvedic drug prepared from mica (which may be an organometallic complex of mica). Mica mainly contains the silicates of iron, magnesium and aluminum[34]. In recent years silicon and silicates have been used for the treatment of diseases. Howard and Lloyed[35] have shown that the behavior of silicate nanocolloid as free radical scavenger *in vivo*. Abhrak bhasma might be behaving as free radical scavenger and reducing ER damage.

Thus from the present study is clear that Abhrak bhasma protects liver and kidney against CCl_4 toxicity and high lipid turnover occurs during CCl_4 toxicity.

References

1. Robinson D S, The clearing factor lipase and its actions in the transport of fatty acids between the blood and the tissues, in *Advances In Lipid Res, ed. by Raoletti & D Kritchevsky* (academic press, New York) *1* (1963) 133 – 182

2. Guyton A C, Lipid and protein metabolism, in *Human Physiology and Mechanisms of Disease.* Published by W B Sounders Company, a division of Harcourt Brace and company Philadelphia

3. Rizack M A, Activation of epinephrine – sensitive lipolytic activity from adipose tissue by adenosine 3,5 – phosphate, *J Biol Chem, 239* (1964) 392-395

4. Vaughan M, Berger J E and Steiberg D, Hormone sensitive lipase and monoglyceride lipase activities in adipose tissue, *J Biol Chem, 239* (1964) 401-409

5. Eagan J J, Greenberg A S, Chans M K, Wek S A, Moose M C and Londas C Mechanism of hormone stimulated lipolysis in adipocytes : translocation of hormone

sensitive lipase to the lipid storsse droplet, *Proc Natl Acad Sci USA*, 89 (1992) 8531-8541

6. Mahadevan S & tappel A L, Lysosomal lipases of rat liver and kidney, *J Biol Chem*, 243 (1968) 2849-2854

7. Hayase K and Tappel A L, Specificity and other properties of lysomal lipase of rat liver, *J Biol Chem* 245 (1970) 169-75

8. Colbeau A; Cuault F & Vignais P M, Characterization and subcellular localization of lipase activities in rat liver cell. Comparison with phospholipase A, *Biochemie*, 56 (1974) 275-288

9. Colbeau A; Nago-tri H; Chaber J and Vignais P M, Are monoglyceride lipase, triglyceride lipase and phospolipase A of rat liver microsomes different entities?, *Biochemie*, 59 (1977) 517-26

10. Anderson R and Sando G N, Cloning and expression of cDNA encoding human lysosomal acid lipase / cholesteryl ester hydrolase. Similarities to gastric and lingual lipases *J Biol Chem*, 226 (1991) 22479-22484

11. Assmann G; Krauss R M; Fredrickson D S; & Levy R I, Characterization, subcellular localization, and partial purification of a heparin-released triglyceride lipase from rat liver, *J Biol Chem*, 248 (1973) 1992-1999

12. Ikeda Y Okamura K and Fujii S, Purification and characterization of rat liver monoglycerol lipase in comparison to other esterases, *Biochim Biophys Acta*, 488 (1977) 128-139

13. Devarshi P; Kanase A: Kanase R; Mane S; Patil S and Varute A T Effect of mandur bhasma on lipolytic activities of liver, kidney and adipose tissue of albino rat during CCl_4 induced acute hepatic injury, *J Biosci*, 10 (1986) 227-234

14. Patil S, Kanase A & Varute A T, Effect of hepatoprotective ayurvedic drugs on lypolytic activities during CCl_4 induced acute hepatic injury in albino rats 31 (1993) 265-269

15. Patil S, Kanase A & Varute A T, Effect of hepatoprotective ayurvedic drugs on lipases following CCl_4 induced hepatic injury in rats *Indian J Exp Biol*, 27 (1989) 955-958

16. Roullier C H, Experimental toxic injury of the liver. *In The Liver, Ed by C H Roullier* [Academic Press New York] vol. 2, [1963] pp. 335

17. Caponnetto A, Randinone R, Zunin P, Alpha-linolenic acid and its metabolic deriva-

tives in the tissues of rats treated with CCl4, *Boll Soc Ital Biol Sper, 60* (1984) 1997-2002

18. Dobrynina O V, Migushina V L, Shatinina S Z & Boldanova N B, Use of Phospholipids to repair rat liver membranes during carbon tetrachloride poisoning, *Biull Eksp Biol Med 104* (1987) 301-303

19. Nakata R, Tsukamoto I, Nanme M, Makino S, Miyoshi M & Kajo S, Alpha adrenergic regulation of the activity of thymidylate synthetase and thymidine kinase during liver regeneration after partial hepatectomy, *Eur J Pharmacol 114* (1985) 355-60

20. Buwa S, Patil S, Kulkarni P H & Kanase A, Evaluation of hepatoprotective actions of Abhrak bhasma in albino rats after the induction of hepatitis by the single dose of CCl_4 *Deerghayu International, 15* (1999) 160-162

21. Matsumura S, Matsuda T, Matsuo M, Kumon A, Sudo K and Nishizuka Y, Studies on triglyceride lipases from rat adipose tissue, *J Biochem, 80* (1976) 351-359

22. Itaya K, A more sensitive and stable calorimetric determination of free fatty acids in blood, *J Lipid Res, 18* (1977) 663-665

23. Lowry O H, Rosebrough N J, Farr A L & Randall R J, Protein measurement with Folin Phenol reagent, *J Biol Chem 193* (1951) 265-275

24. Tornqvist H & Belfrage P, Determination of protein in adipose tissue extracts, *J Lipid Res. 17* (1976) 542-545

25. Agarwal Y P, Statistical methods, concepts, applications and computation (Sterling Publishers Pvt. Ltd., New Delhi) (1990)

26. Elias H and Sherrick J C, in Morphology of the liver, Pub by Academic Press New York and London (1968)

27. Mehendale H M, Hepatic toxicity, in Modern Toxicology vol I Ed by Gupta B V and Salunke D K, Pub by M D Metropolian Book Co. Pvt Ltd., N S Marg, New Delhi (1985)

28. Plaa G L, Chlorinated methames and liver injury : Highlights of the past 50 years. *Annu Rev Pharmacol Toxicol 40* (2000) 34-64

29. Kanase R, Patil S & Kanase A, Effect of hepatoprotective ayurvedic drugs on lysosomal enzymes during hepatic injury induced by single dose of CCl_4. *Ind J Exp Biol, 32* (1994) 328-332

30. Kato H and Nakayawa Y, The effect of carbon tetrachloride on the enzymatic

hydrolysis of cellular triacylglycerol in adult rat hepatocytes in primary monolayer culture. *Bichem Pharmacol, 36* (1987) 1807-1814

31. Teng M H & Kaplan A, Purification and properties of rat liver lysosomal lipase, *J Biol Chem 249* (1974) 1064-1070

32. Debeer L J; Thomas J; De Schepper P and Mannaerts G P, Lysosomal triacylglycerol lipase and lipolysis in isolated rat hepatocytes, *J Biol Chem, 254* (1979) 8841-8846

33. Slater T F, Lysosomes and experimentally induced tissue injury, in Lysosomes in Biology and Pathology, vol. I ed by J T Dingle & H B Fell Published by North Holland Publishing Company, Amsterdam (1966) 467-488

34. Sharma S Rasa Samuchhaya Published by Motilal Banarasidas, New Delhi [1977] pp. 72-108

35. Howard C H and Lloyd K Presented at the American College of Nutrition Symposium on advances in clinical Nutrition Abstracts of Evaluation studies of Microhydrin-A Functional silicate Nanocolloid (1998)

Table 1_a – Abhrak bhasma mediated variations in the wet weights of liver, kidney and adipose tissue of albino rat during hepatitis induced by single dose of CCl_4

[Values are expressed as mg/g body wt]

Group	Liver	Kidney	Adipose tissue
Normal	33.32 ± 1.68	6.70 ± 0.39	6.79 ± 0.35
CCl_4	39.89 ± 1.92[c]	6.67 ± 0.41[d]	6.33 ± 0.47[a]
CCl_4 + Abhrak bhasma [10mg/kg body wt]	30.63 ± 1.83[a,g]	6.16 ± 0.51[a,c]	6.04 ± 0.33[b,c]
CCl_4 + Abhrak bhasma [20mg/kg body wt]	30.91 ± 2.06[c,h]	6.08 ± 0.43[a,c]	6.06 ± 0.45[b,c]
CCl_4 + Abhrak bhasma [30mg/kg body wt]	30.79 ± 2.18[c,h]	6.18 ± 0.38[a,c]	6.70 ± 0.44[d,f]
CCl_4 + Abhrak bhasma [40mg/kg body wt]	30.52 ± 1.63[c,h]	6.42 ± 0.31[d,g]	7.36 ± 0.52[d,c]

Values are mean ± SE of 8 animals

P Values – a<0.05, b<0.01, c<0.001 & d>0.05
E<0.05, f<0.01, g<0.001 & h>0.05

Table 2 – Effect of Abhrak bhasma on lipolytic enzymes of liver during hepatitis induced By single dose of CCl_4

Group	Acid lipase		Alkaline lipase		Lipoprotein lipase	
	K Units/g tissue	Units/mg protein	K Units/g tissue	Units/mg protein	K Units/g tissue	Units/mg protein
Normal	10.15 ± 3.33	47.34 ± 2.80	19.50 ± 1.27	90.97 ± 3.71	2.50 ± 0.08	11.66 ± 0.58
CCl_4	4.10 ± 1.17[c]	16.10 ± 0.74[c]	08.05 ± 0.42[h,g]	31.62 ± 1.44[c]	6.70 ± 0.39[c]	26.32 ± 1.92[c]
CCl_4 + Abhrak Bhasma [10 mg/kg body wt]	05.20 ± 0.36[c,g]	28.74 ± 1.85[c,g]	10.45 ± 0.41[h,g]	55.22 ± 2.86[c,g]	8.50 ± 0.34[c,f]	46.98 ± 2.88[c,g]
CCl_4 + Abhrak Bhasma [20 mg/kg body wt]	08.65 ± 0.53[b,g]	53.79 ± 2.74[c,g]	15.55 ± 0.73[c,g]	96.60 ± 3.47[a,g]	11.25 ± 0.51[c,g]	69.96 ± 4.27[c,g]
CCl_4 + Abhrak Bhasma [30 mg/kg body wt]	12.50 ± 0.57[b,g]	60.16 ± 2.56[c,g]	17.75 ± 0.94[b,h]	85.43 ± 3.12[a,g]	27.50 ± 1.83[c,g]	132.35 ± 6.35[c,g]
CCl_4 + Abhrak Bhasma [40 mg/kg body wt]	9.00 ± 0.44[a,g]	57.73 ± 2.19[b,g]	19.10 ± 0.85[d,f]	122.51 ± 4.07[c,g]	31.00 ± 2.03[c,g]	198.85 ± 8.00[c,g]

Values are mean ± SE of 8 animals

P values are as in Table 1

Hepatic Disorders

Table 3 – Effect of Abhrak bhasma on lipolytic enzymes of liver during hepatitis induced By single dose of CCl_4

Group	Acid lipase		Alkaline lipase		Lipoprotein lipase	
	K Units/g tissue	Units/mg protein	K Units/g tissue	Units/mg protein	K Units/g tissue	Units/mg protein
Normal	08.60 ± 0.43	67.56 ± 4.09	10.50 ± 0.40	82.48 ± 7.90	16.50 ± 0.071	129.62 ± 6.79
CCl_4	03.60 ± 0.16[c]	29.85 ± 1.16[c]	05.00 ± 0.25[c]	41.46 ± 2.00[c,g]	04.70 ± 0.17[c]	38.97 ± 3.05[c]
CCl_4 + Abhrak Bhasma [10 mg/kg body wt]	06.60 ± 0.33[b,g]	49.29 ± 3.33[c,g]	03.80 ± 0.09[c,g]	28.38 ± 1.04[c,g]	24.10 ± 1.09[c,g]	179.99 ± 8.38[c,g]
CCl_4 + Abhrak Bhasma [20 mg/kg body wt]	07.75 ± 0.47[a,g]	52.58 ± 4.18[c,g]	06.65 ± 0.41[c,g]	45.12 ± 3.26[c,c]	25.14 ± 1.63[c,g]	170.67 ± 7.73[c,g]
CCl_4 + Abhrak Bhasma [30 mg/kg body wt]	16.00 ± 0.92[c,g]	66.33 ± 3.92[d,g]	08.00 ± 0.39[c,g]	33.17 ± 1.64[c,g]	23.56 ± 0.96[c,g]	97.66 ± 5.07[c,g]
CCl_4 + Abhrak Bhasma [40 mg/kg body wt]	18.50 ± 1.07[c,g]	120.05 ± 5.48[c,g]	10.05 ± 0.49[a,g]	65.22 ± 3.27[c,g]	24.45 ± 1.45[c,g]	158.45 ± 6.14[c,g]

Values are mean ± SE of 8 animals

P values are as in Table 1

Table 4 – Effect of Abhrak bhasma on lipolytic enzymes of liver during hepatitis induced By single dose of CCl_4

Group	Acid lipase		Alkaline lipase		Lipoprotein lipase		Hormone sensitive lipase	
	K Units / g Tissue	Units / mg Protein	K Units / g Tissue	Units / mg Protein	K Units / g Tissue	Units / mg Protein	K Units / g Tissue	Units / mg Protein
Normal	2.10 ± 0.06	39.18 ± 1.74	4.65 ± 0.20	86.75 ± 4.31	2.50 ± 0.12	46.64 ± 2.37	8.10 ± 0.44	151.12 ± 6.38
CCl_4	1.60 ± 1.04[c]	31.84 ± 1.46[b]	12.50 ± 0.55[c]	248.76 ± 14.84[c]	26.90 ± 0.87[c]	535.32 ± 28.00[c]	38.25 ± 12.05[c]	761.79 ± 34.00[c]
CCl_4 + Abhrak Bhasma [10 mg/kg body wt]	4.25 ± 0.21[c-g]	105.72 ± 4.81[c-g]	18.00 ± 0.86[c-g]	447.76 ± 21.51[c-g]	24.40 ± 1.06[c-c]	606.97 ± 40.28[c-g]	23.75 ± 2.03[c-g]	590.71 ± 31.31[c-g]
CCl_4 + Abhrak Bhasma [20 mg/kg body wt]	4.00 ± 0.13[c-g]	49.74 ± 1.92[c-g]	15.05 ± 0.67[c-l]	187.14 ± 9.15[c-g]	20.70 ± 0.84[c-g]	257.40 ± 12.41[c-g]	14.05 ± 0.94[c-g]	174.71 ± 9.03[c-g]
CCl_4 + Abhrak Bhasma [30 mg/kg body wt]	3.05 ± 0.17[c-g]	46.02 ± 2.33[c-g]	8.75 ± 0.48[c-g]	132.02 ± 6.51[c-g]	16.25 ± 0.77[c-g]	245.17 ± 14.00[c-g]	11.90 ± 0.48[c-g]	179.54 ± 7.77[c-g]
CCl_4 + Abhrak Bhasma [40 mg/kg body wt]	2.35 ± 0.15[a-g]	43.84 ± 3.10[b-g]	6.88 ± 0.36[c-g]	128.00 ± 5.13[c-g]	12.75 ± 0.53[c-g]	237.87 ± 10.89[c-g]	6.00 ± 0.43[c-g]	111.94 ± 5.86[b-g]

Values are mean ± SE of 8 animals

P values are as in Table 1

Hepatic Disorders

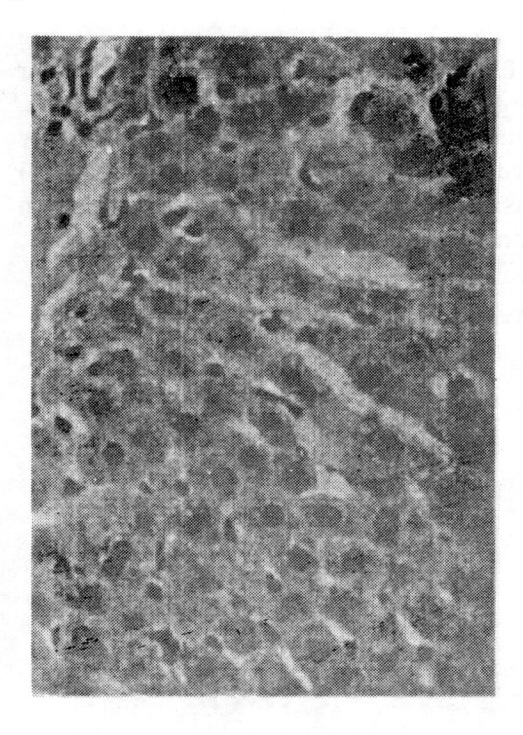

Fig. 1 : Normal rat : Centrolobular region shows normal hepatic cords, hepatocytes, sinusoids, bile canaliculi, Kupffer cells X 250

Fig. 2 : CCl_4 treated rat : Centrolobular necrosis. Zone rich in the hepatocytes with vacuolar necrosis, obliterated bile canaliculi, sinusoids, arrested Kupffer cells in necrotic region X 250

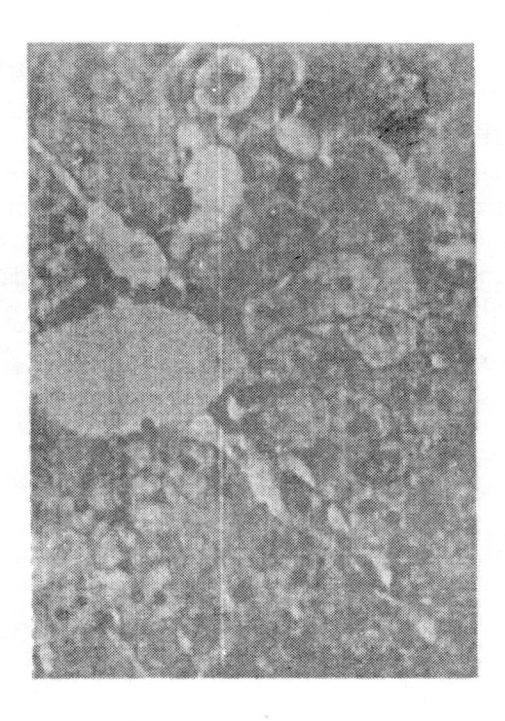

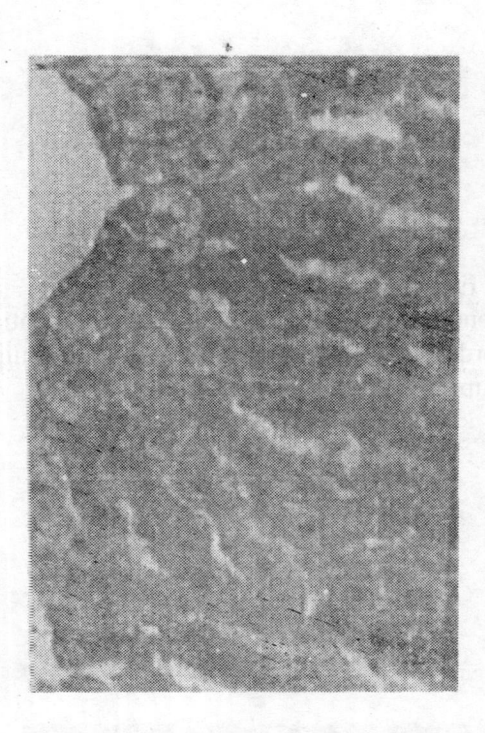

Fig. 3 : CCl$_4$ + 10 mg Abhrak bhasma treated rat : **Centrolobular region**. Note reduction necrotic area, increased number of hepatocytes, partially protected hepatocytes and bile canaliculi visible in some regions. Sinusoids cleared in some region X 250

Fig. 4 : CCl$_4$ + 20 mg Abhrak bhasma treated rat : centrolobular region. Note normalized picture of centrolobular region. Fully protected hepatocytes, normal sinusoids, clear bile canaliculi, Kupffer cell and sinusoidal cells cleared X 250.

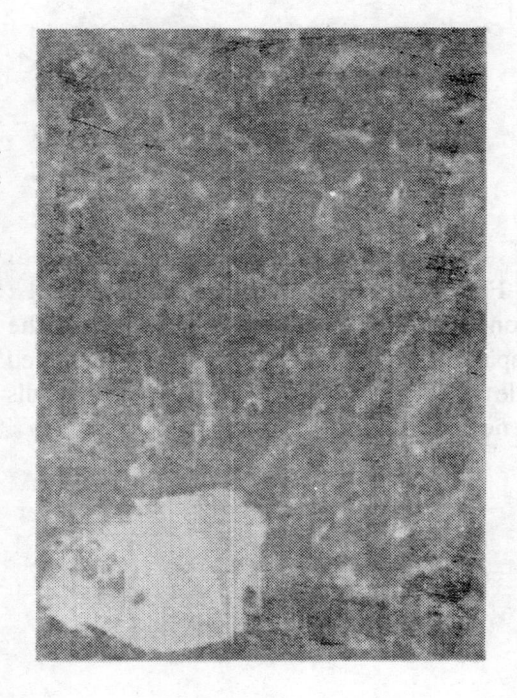

Hepatic Disorders

Kumari Kalpa Ghansar Tablets Research With Microscopic High Resolution Blood Morphology Test (Peripheral Live Blood Analysis) In Chronic Fatigue Syndrome (CFS)

Dr. E.B.S. Premdani,

Introduction :

In this case of research I would like to discuss mainly the matter of toxins (known in Ayurveda as AMA) and parasites in the blood in relation with **Kumari Kalpa**.

Microscopic Peripheral High Blood Resolution Morphology Test (also known as Live Blood Analysis) through the use of the BVPM (Bradford variable projection microscope) is a unique and innovative cost effective way to assess the amount and general location of oxidative processes within the body.

Peripheral Blood assessment can determine processes within the body, as well as hormones, erythrocytes, leukocytes, enzymes, fungus (Candida Albicans), parasites, toxins, bacteria's, and other by-products of biological stress, etc.

Spicules

Spicules are being seen in Live blood analysis with dark-field as well as phase-contrast microcopy as spikes, needle-like structures.

According to the Bradford Research institute they are mutated platelets, forming these needle-like projections, which is an indication of Liver-stress.

The German Prof. Dr. Günther Enderlein called them filiten. According to him this is a sign of endobiosis (congestion where the blood cells are infected with parasitic growth forms in which the Liver is very much stressed). So, both Bradford and Enderlein claim the spicules to be an indication of Liver-stress.

This stress may be the result of excessive use of drugs, chemotherapy, radiation, alcohol, viral infections, bacterial infections, parasitic infections or a slowing down of the Liver function due to fat build-up, etc.

Hepatic Disorders

Ayurveda and spicules.

With the knowledge of our beautiful science called Ayurveda, I observed these spicules for more then 14 years. To me these spicules are nothing more than what is called in Ayurveda as AMA (undigested food rests) also indicating Liver stress and low Liver agni.

I used **Kumari Kalpa** in more then hundreds of cases of Chronic Fatigue Syndrome patients.

In short, Chronic Fatigue patients suffer from the following symptoms : severe fatigue, Candida yeast infection with swollen glands, hypoglycaemia, muscle aching, cramps, diarrhoea, bloating, headaches, intermittent spiking fevers, nightsweats, sensitivities to light or dark, cold or heat, body clothes, bed clothes, food, drink, the air conditioning, shampoos, lacquers, perfumes, lack of sleep – or too much sleep – plus short-term memory loss, mood swings, depression, allergies to many things like foods, pollen, synthetic chemicals, provoking rashes, runny noses, red eyes, puffy eye bags, sleep disturbances, pains in the joints and bones.

If, in their case, mononucleosis, hepatitis, the ARC stage of AIDS, secondary syphilis, pre-menstrual syndrome, hypoglycaemia, mercury poisoning from dental amalgams and thyroid problems have been eliminated as cause, they might be called " post-viral syndrome " or even " myalgic encephalomyelitis " (ME) patients.

Though Chronic Fatigue is not a known disease in India, I believe that Ayurveda can do a lot for these patients, as I do in my clinic in the Netherlands with great help of my Ayurvedic research professor P.H. Kulkarni.

Liver diseases :

Liver, the most active organ of the human body, is also the most vulnerable to disorders and damages due to various exogenous and endogenous Hepato-toxins.

Being the largest gland of the body it secretes about 600-800 ml of bile daily. Besides its secretary and excretory functions, it also controls the numerous metabolic functions, such as, metabolism of fats, proteins, minerals, carbohydrates, biotransformation, etc. It also plays a major role during inflammation, immune reaction etc.

The disorders associated with the Liver are numerous and varied. Liver disorders may be classified as acute or chronic hepatitis (inflammatory Liver diseases), hepatitis (non-inflammatory disorders) and Liver cirrhosis (degenerative disorders resulting in fibrosis of the Liver). The Primary event of the most Liver pathogenesis being the Liver cell necrosis.

The major causes of various Liver diseases like hepatitis, cirrhosis and jaundice is due to contamination with the virus A or B, excessive alcohol consumption and drug abuse.

Hepatic Disorders

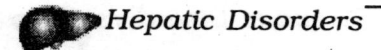

Liver and Chronic Fatigue syndrome

In all Chronic Fatigue patients I have observed Liver stress, seen as spicules (filiten, AMA) in peripheral blood assessment. Because the body of a Chronic Fatigue patient is complete burned out, it is no wonder all the organs are burned out as well. In Live Blood Analysis I also see besides spicules, rouleaux formation (this is where red blood cells adhere to each other to form a " stack of coins ") due to hyper-proteinemia in the bloodstream, protein linking (this is due to low agni in the small intestines).

Because the Liver is so congested with AMA, it presses it out the Liver Srota's as spicules (AMA) in the blood-circulation.

Most of Chronic Fatigue patients who were suffering from pain in the Liver area found total relief after using *Kumari Kalpa*.

Use of *Kumari Kalpa* in the Netherlands :

Most of the doctors and naturopaths in the Netherlands stopped prescribing their homeopathic or other hepatic medicines after start using *Kumari Kalpa*. Many of them are testing *Kumari Kalpa* through electro-acupuncture machines like Vega and Mora.

Dr. Hulda Clark

According to the American Dr. Hulda Clark, writer of *Cure of all Cancer*, claims that cancer can be caused by a parasite, the human intestinal fluke called *fasciolopsis buskii*. If it establishes in the Liver, it causes cancer. The Kupffer cells in the Liver, which are reticuloendothelial cells capable of phagocytizing bacteria, parasites etc. are responsible for killing the *fasciolopsis buskii*.

Kumari Kalpa helps the Liver in protecting against these parasites. Treating patients with parasite in blood I observed a tremendous decrease of parasite by treating the patients with *Kumari Kalpa*.

Clinical trials

By giving the dose of *Kumari Kalpa* 2 times 2 tablets daily for one month there is a decrease of the spicules of 50 %. After two moths use there is a decrease of spicules of 90 %. After three moths we see a total 100 % decrease of Spicules.

Though I selected to detoxify and strengthen the Liver by supplying *Kumari Kalpa* in cases of Chronic Fatigue syndrome patients, I also saw a decrease in Cholesterol in Hypercholesterolemia patients as well in the high Liver enzymes SGOT, SGPT, g -GT, Alkaline phosphatase.

Hepatic Disorders

Observations :

Table : Decrease of Spicules in 100 chronic fatigue patients.

Chronic fatigue Patients	Decrease Spicules after 1 month use of KK	Decrease Spicules after 2 month use of KK	Decrease Spicules after 3 month use of KK
2 CFS patients	40 %	65 %	75 %
3 CFS patients	40 %	70 %	80 %
5 CFS patients	45 %	80 %	90 %
6 CFS patients	45 %	85 %	95 %
84 CFS patients	50 %	90 %	100 %

Composition of Kumari Kalpa Ghansar tablets:

- Kumari Ghansar (Aloe vera)
- Guduchi (Tinospora cordifolia)
- Terminalia chebula (Haritaki)
- Chitrak (Plumbago zeylanica)
- Pushkarmool (Saussurea lappa)
- Twak taila (Cinnamomum zeylanicum)
- Bruhat (Solanum indicum)
- Shaliparni (Desmodium gangeticum)
- Agnimanth (Clerodendron phlomoidis)
- Patala (Stereospermum sauveolens)
- Lavang Bhasma (Caryophyllus aromaticus)
- Ghambari (Gmelina arborea)
- Bibhitaki (Terminalia belerica)
- Katuka (Picrorrhiza kurrua)
- Chavya (Piper chaba)
- Punarnava (Boerhaavia diffusa)
- Kartatshringi (Pistacia integerima)
- kantakari (Solanum xanthocarpum)
- Pushniparni (Uraria picta)
- Jatiphala Taila (Myristica fragruns)
- Bilva (Aegle marmelos)
- Tintuk (Oroxylum indicum)
- Vasa (Adhatoda vasica)
- Gokshur (Tribulus terrestris)

Hepatic Disorders

Before treatment :

Test results in High Resolution Blood Morfology (Live-Blood-Analysis) before treatment with ***Kumari Kalpa***. A lot of spicules or AMA (indication of Liver stress) and Rouleau Formation (indication of poor digestion) and Parasites.

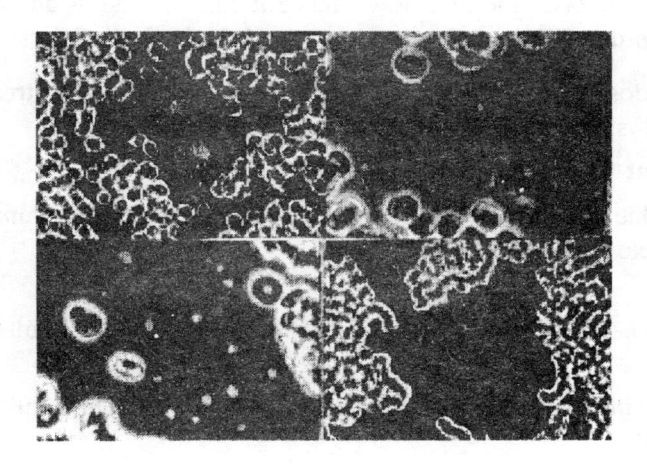

After treatment :

Test results after treatment with ***Kumari Kalpa***. No spicules and Rouleau Formation and parasites to be seen in the blood-sample.

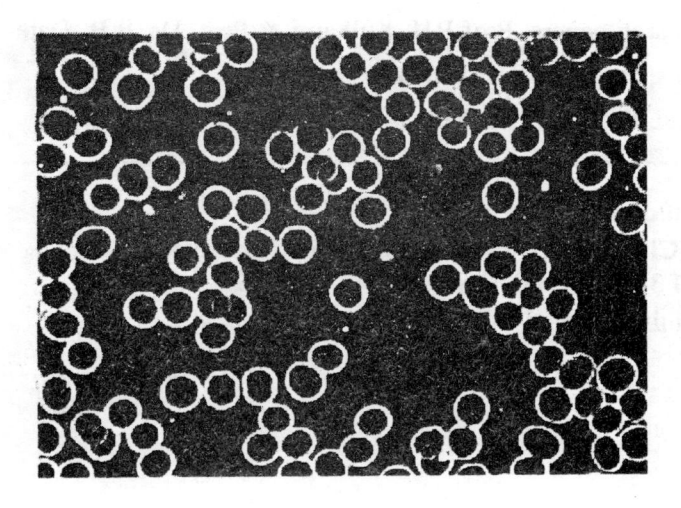

Conclusion :

So far I experienced that Kumari Kalpa showed the best results in decreasing the spicules (indication of Liver stress), Rouleau formation and parasites in the blood.

Kumari Kalpa as a Ayurvedic polyherbal formulation, not only aids, tones and strengthens the Liver, but also increases the bile flow. Hence it can be used as an herbal remedy for various hepatic disorders like hepatitis, hepatosis, and alcoholic disorders.

Increase of the dose of Kumari Kalpa doesn't show extra effect in treatment. The best dose I experienced is 2 tablets two times per day after meal.

Acknowledgement :

My thanks are due to Prof. P.H. Kulkarni and Ayurved Rasashala, Pune. My thanks are also due to Institute of Indian Medicine.

Referenties :

1. Bradford research institute, chronic fatigue syndrome, Michael L. Culbert, Dr. R. Bradford.
2. The examination into darkfield diagnostics according to Prof. Dr. Günther Enderlein, Dr.Frantz Arnoul,
3. Clinical Assessment of Kumari Kalpa Ghansar Tabs in anorexia, Prof. Dr. Kulkarni & Prof. B.B. Date, Deerghayu international.
4. Fundamentals of Ayurvedic Medicine, 7th edition, Vaidya Bhagwan Dash.
5. Prakruti, Your Ayurvedic Constitution, Dr. Robert E. Svoboda
6. Ayurveda Philosofy, Prof. Dr. P.H. Kulkarni
7. Ayurveda Research papers, Prof P.H. Kulkarni & Prof. Dr. B.B. Date
8. Ayurveda Herbs, Prof. Dr. P.H. Kulkarni
9. Ayurveda Nidan, Prof. Dr. P.H. Kulkarni

Dr. E. B. S. Premdani
Premdani Health Clinic, Rijksstraatweg 195, 3956 CM Leersum,
Holland, Tel : +31 343 46 13 00, Fax : +31 343 46 01 39
E-mail : e.premdani@hetnet.nl

Hepatic Disorders

Liver Cancer Treatment As It Stands Today

Dr. Koppikar C.B.

Cancer of the liver can be primary – one that originates in the liver itself, or secondary - a spread from other organs. Liver cancer was considered to be the end of the road for the patient. However, with improvements in surgical techniques and the advent of new modalities of treatment this assumption is no longer true. Newer strategies are being developed the world over which aim at cure as well as prolonging and improving the quality of life of the patients. Treatment of liver tumors is a dynamic process, and various treatments are now used singly or in combination to achieve optimum results.

We have joined this quest of seeking new treatments to improve the quality of life of liver cancer patients and have introduced treatments like Hepatic Intra-arterial Chemotherapy, Cryosurgery, etc along with the usual liver resections which cut away the affected part of the liver.

Liver resection

Whenever possible an attempt is made to remove the tumor. Only when the tumor is unresectable, the other modalities are used. Resection includes major excision of the liver parenchyma such as extended left or right hepatectomies and minor ones like segmentectomies and wide local excisions

Treatment of liver tumors is a dynamic process. Various modalities are used singly or in combination to achieve optimum result, which needs a specialized team of doctors

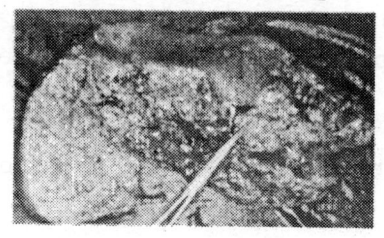

Intra-arterial Hepatic Chemotherapy

In this, chemotherapy is delivered directly into the liver by surgically placing a catheter in the hepatic artery, which is known to supply blood to the tumor preferentially. Drugs are delivered via the catheter directly into the artery that channels most of it to the tumor. These concentrated drugs act more effectively on the cancer than the conventional chemotherapy. Further, the drugs do not affect the normal liver cells, as well as the other systems of the body resulting in very few side effects. Thus this treatment improves the quality of life, and increases the life span of such patients.

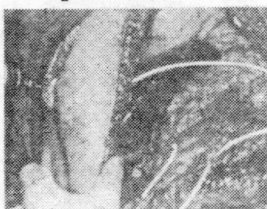

Cryosurgery

Cryosurgery is a novel technique that supplements the surgeon's blade with a specialized apparatus. Here Liquid nitrogen is circulated through the apparatus, which generates very low temperatures at its probe. This probe is then inserted in the tumor thereby freezing it. This process is repeated twice, thus getting rid of the tumor. This procedure ensures minimal bleeding when compared to conventional surgery, and markedly improves the curable rate of unresectable liver tumors. This method of treatment is presently new to India

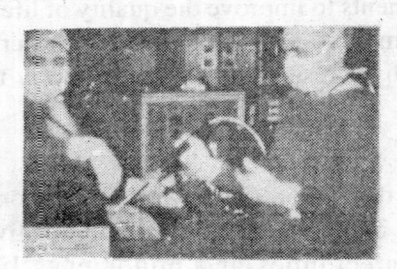

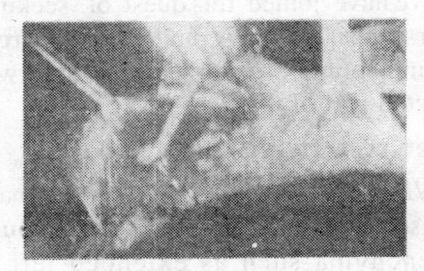

There are still other modalities of treatments available for advanced cases wherein the tumor is attacked by either direct injection of alcohol or by embolisation of the hepatic artery.

Even after so many modalities being currently available the scenario of liver cancers is still very grim. The problems peculiar to the Indian context are

1. Delay in diagnosis

2. Lack of awareness amongst patients as well as doctors about possible treatment

Hepatic Disorders

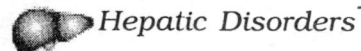

options

3. Presence of diseased liver along with the tumor [liver cirrhosis]
4. Financial constraints

To conclude, liver cancer though treatable poses a tough challenge to us and it is only determination and perseverance on the part of the patient and his family as well as the treating team of doctors that the battle can be won. The silver lining in the dark cloud is that a large number of patients have fared reasonably well thanks to the multidisciplinary approach the details of which will be presented along with slides and videoclips.

Dr. Koppikar C. B.
38, Banu Apts., Dastur Meher Road, Camp, Pune – 411 001
Tel : 020 – 6219080 Fax : 020 – 6129037 E-mail koppiker@hotmail.com

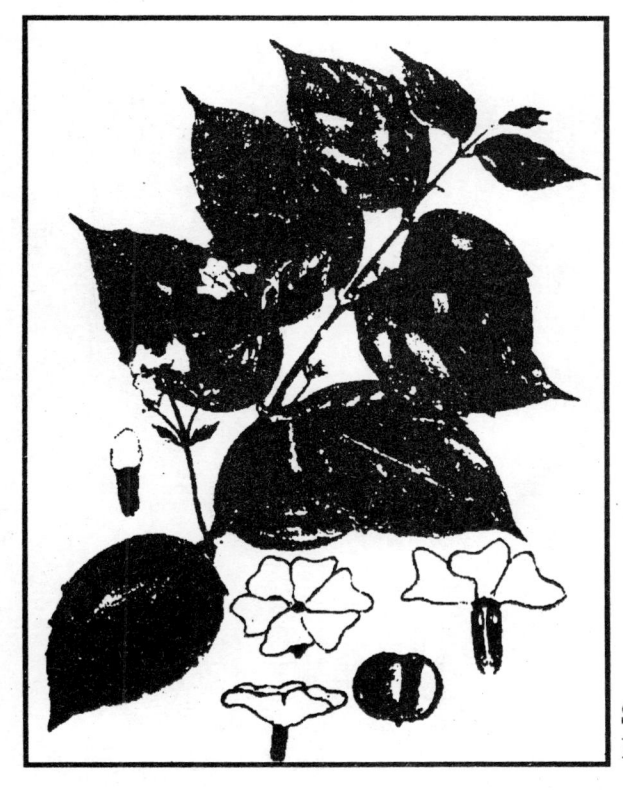

Sanskrit Name : Parijatak
Latin Name : Nyctanthus arbortristis

Hepatic Disorders

Chronic Hepatitis B Virus Infection

Dr Vinay K Thorat

There are about three hundred and twenty million people chronically infected by the hepatitis B virus (HBV) worldwide. Since its postulated existence as an antigen in Australian Aborigines in 1965 it has continued to occupy center stage in hepatology and community medicine worldwide.

Fate of HBV on entering the body.

Once HBV enters the human body by the parenteral route it attaches itself to the hepatocyte by means of a receptor. Once this happens the viral DNA i.e. HBV DNA enters the hepatocyte. The DNA, which has codes for the various viral proteins as well as the enzymes, needed for replication of the HBV DNA itself. The replicating virus and the viral proteins gain access to

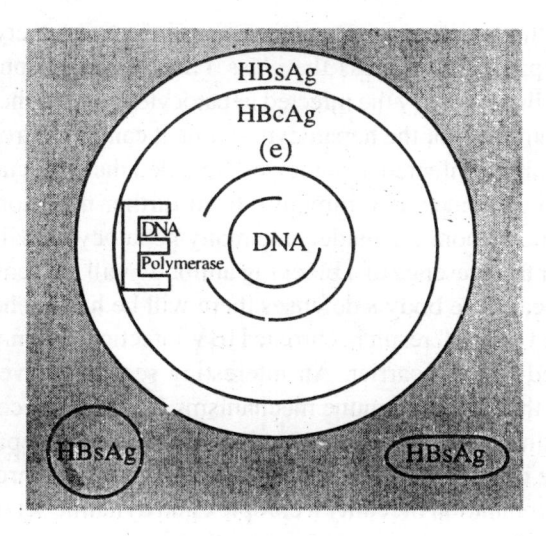

Fig. 1 A diagrammatic representation of HBV

the blood stream by destruction of infected hepatocytes. As the various viral proteins enter the blood stream an antibody response is mounted against these proteins. Identification of viral antigens and the respective antibodies forms the cornerstone of identifying the various stages of HBV infection in a given patient. Finally the viral DNA integrates itself into the hepatocyte DNA a step which precedes the development of hepatocellular carcinoma (HCC). The principal viral proteins produced are the hepatitis B surface antigen (HbsAg), the core protein which envelopes the DNA, the DNA polymerase, reverse transcriptase and viral DNA itself. The e antigen is a by-product of the core protein, and is found in the blood. A close look at the structure of HBV helps understand these various fractions much better (Fig 1)

Fate of the infected hepatocyte

All the various types of HBV infection related responses by the body essentially depend on how the body's immune system handles the HBV infection (Fig 2).

HBV DNA IN THE HEPATOCYTE

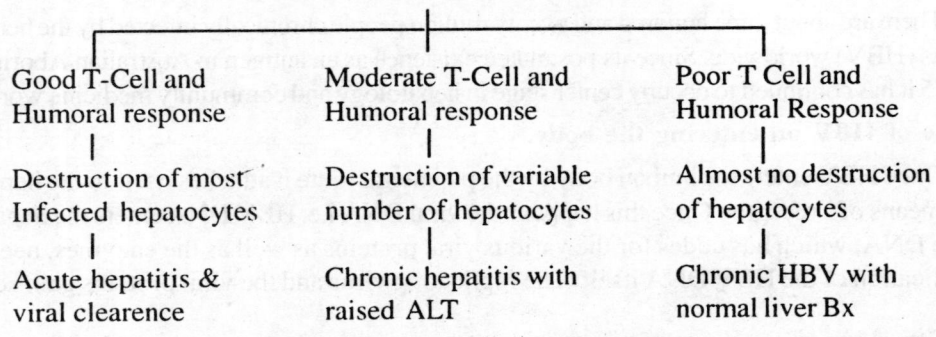

Good T-Cell and Humoral response	Moderate T-Cell and Humoral response	Poor T Cell and Humoral Response
Destruction of most Infected hepatocytes	Destruction of variable number of hepatocytes	Almost no destruction of hepatocytes
Acute hepatitis & viral clearance	Chronic hepatitis with raised ALT	Chronic HBV with normal liver Bx

Once the virus enters the hepatocyte in acute primary infection ninety five percent of the times all the infected hepatocytes express the class 1 HLA antigen on their surface. This allows the body's killer cells to identify the infected hepatocytes and kill them. This liberates the virus from the protected environs of the hepatocyte so that it can be destroyed by humoral and other mechanisms. Since all the infected hepatocytes are killed there is acute hepatitis followed usually by complete viral clearance and immunity from further infection. However in some patients where the immune response is inadequate many hepatocytes will fail to show up the MHC class one antigen or the presence of a blocking antibody will prevent their destruction. If almost all hepatocytes escape the body's defenses there will be hardly hepatocytes killed by the bodies killer T cells and this will result in chronic HBV infection with no chronic hepatitis on liver biopsy, the so called healthy carrier. An interesting scenario develops if some of the hepatocytes are killed by the bodied immune mechanisms while others continue to harbor the virus and infect regenerating cells. This results in a limited number of hepatocytes being killed at any given point of time but without total viral clearance leading to chronic active hepatitis. Though this is a simple explanation in reality a complex and dynamic set of both viral and host factors actually determine the outcome of HBV infection.

Hepatic Disorders

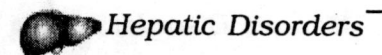

Risk of chronicity in HBV infection.

A majority of acute HBV infections will clear by six months. However in neonates the chances of chronicity is ninety percent in neonates and 30 percent in those between one and five years of age.

Indicators of chronic HBV infection.

The indicators of chronic HBV infection can be either clinical, biochemical, immunological or histological. Clinical indicators include the presence of jaundice with fever or fatigue and weight loss with or without edema, ascites, spider naevi, palmer erythema and hepatosplenomegaly for more than six months. Biochemically elevated transaminases for more than six months indicate chronic hepatitis. The presence of IgG anti HB core antibody along with HbsAg or the presence of HbsAg for over six months indicates chronic HBV infection. Liver biopsies may show fibrosis a hallmark of chronicity. Presence of bridging and piecemeal necrosis though highly suggestive of chronic hepatitis is not diagnostic. The chronically infected patient can evolve into any of the following clinical situations

HBV without significant liver disease

Chronic hepatitis

Cirrhosis

Hepatocellular Carcinoma

HBV related Immune Complex disorders

Serodiagnosis of HBV infection.

Very early in HBV infection there is liberation of viral proteins into the body. This leads to an IgM response and a late IgG response to some viral proteins, which help identify the phase of HBV infection.

The following tables indicate the presence of various HBV related antigens and antibodies in various HBV related conditions.

HBsAg	HBV infection Acute/Chronic
HBeAg	High levels of replication
Anti-HBe	Low levels of replication
Anti-HBc (IgM)	Recent HBV infection
Anti-HBc (IgG)	Recovered or Chronic HBV
Anti-HBs	Immunity to HBV infection
Anti-HBc (IgG) & Anti HBs	Past HBV infection
Anti-HBc (IgG) & HBsAg	Chronic HBV infection

Hepatic Disorders

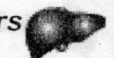

Hence the various markers in the various phases of HBV infection would be as follows

<u>Acute HBV Hepatitis</u>

Early phase	HBsAg, IgM Anti HBc
Window phase	IgM Anti HBc only
Recovered phase	Anti HBs, IgG Anti-HBc

<u>Chronic HBV Hepatitis</u>

Replicative phase	HBsAg, IgG Anti-HBc, HBeAg, HBV DNA
Non (low) replicative	HBsAg, IgG Anti-HBc, Anti HBe
Precore mutant	HBsAg, Anti-HBe, IgG Anti HBc, HBV DNA

It is also important to understand HBV DNA assays when planning treatment. PCR detects 1-10 copies per ml and should be used only as research tool. No one is certain of the significance of such low levels of HBV infection in clinical practice. For clinical use two methods are used for DNA assay. Branched DNA assay detects 10000 copies /ml and is more sensitive than molecular hybridization which detects up to 100000 copies per ml. For all practical purposes if DNA is not detected by either of these methods its a low replicative phase and no treatment is needed. Levels of DNA in HBV infected patients usually reported by these assays as expressed in picograms per milliliter are 10 to 200 pg./ml.

Using these markers we are now in a position to determine which patients we should treat and which patients need follow up.

Wild and mutant viruses HBV.

The hepatitis B virus exists not only as the wild variety by also acquires many mutant forms. These mutants tend to present with atypical serological features and may be drug resistant. The wild type of HBV has genotypes A-F with the major determinant 'a' is common. A representation of the HBV genome is shown in Fig 2.

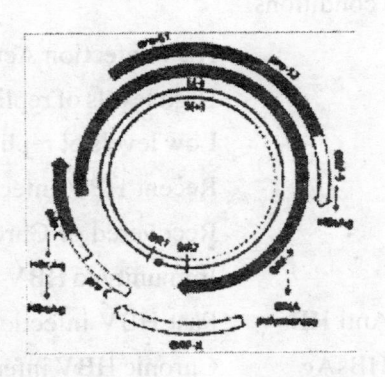

Fig 2. The Genome of HBV

Hepatic Disorders

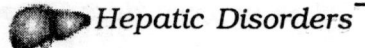

Mutant HBV viruses arise when there is mutation in any of the amino acid sequences of the four partially overlapping regions of the HBV genome which are as follows

1. pre-S/S gene codes the envelope protein.
2. pre-C/C gene codes e Ag and core proteins
3. P gene codes the DNA polymerase & reverse transcriptase
4. X gene

A list of the commonly found mutants is given below

Pre-core region

G-A at nucleotide 1896 is the most extensively found mutant

G-A at nucleotide (nt) 1899

Core promoter region

A-T at nt 1762 & G-A at nt 1764

S gene

Gly-Arg at codon 145

P gene (polymerase and reverse transcriptase)

Lamivudine induced M-V/I at YMDD(a highly conserved locus of P gene) codon 552

L-M at codon 528

Famcyclovir induced mutation L-M at codon 528.

Drug induced mutations lead to drug resistance

Clinically some mutants may cause a more severe disease. Atypical serological features may be present.

HBeAg negative cases with high ALT and necrosis on liver biopsy i.e. active replication is found in many cases. HBsAg negative but HBV DNA positive serology may occur. Mutation at amino acid 145 in the 'a' determinant may cause vaccine escape after apparently successful vaccination Precore mutants tend to be Interferon resistant and P gene drug mutants are resistant to oral antiviral agents.

Treatment of chronic HBV

It is now generally agreed that patients with high ALT who are HbeAg positive or HBV DNA positive and who have necro-inflammatory changes on liver biopsy should receive some form of treatment with either Interferon or antiviral agents. Patients with normal ALT but who are HBV DNA positive and HbeAg positive do not respond to interferon and there may be role for antiviral agents or other approaches in this group. Further in the absence of raised ALT and negative HBV DNA and HbeAg treatment is not required. A broad recommendation of treatment guidelines is given below.

Guidelines for treatment in chronic HBV.

HBeAg	HBVDNA	ALT	TREATMENT
+	+	Normal	IFN ineffective, ? Antivirals
+	+	Raised	IFN
-	+	Raised	IFN maybe, Antivirals ?
-	-	Normal	No treatment required
+/-	+	Cirrhosis	Compensated-IFN,
			Early Decompensation Low dose IFN, ? Antivirals
			Advanced decompensation Antivirals
			Other experimental therapies
+/-	-	Cirrhosis	Observe

(+ present, - absent, IFN Interferon)

The goals of antiviral therapy are sustained suppression of HBV replication. Serologically this means that the HBV DNA should be undetectable in serum and there should be Hbe Ag to Anti HBe seroconversion

and preferably a HBsAg to Anti HBs seroconversion. Remission of liver disease must also be achieved with normalisation of ALT levels and decreased necroinflammation in the liver on biopsy. This will usually translate into an improved clinical outcome with decreased progression to cirrhosis, hepatocellular carcinoma and increased survival.

Several treatment approaches are currently being evaluated for chronic HBV and a summary of these is presented below.

Interferon

Antiviral agents viz. Lamivudine Famcyclovir, Adefovir, Lobucavir, Gancyclovir

Immunomodulatory therapy which can be non-HBV Specific like Interlukin, Thymosin or HBV specific

Like PreS/S peptide vaccine, DNA vaccines and adoptive immunity transfer. Novel Anti viral approaches like targeted delivery of antivirals, Antisense oligonucleotides and Ribozymes

Hepatic Disorders

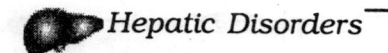

may hold the key to higher rates of eradication of infection.

Clinically however only two types of agents are in extensive use and these are interferons and the antiviral agent Lamivudine with or without famcyclovir.

Interferons are naturally occurring substances which have both immunomodulatory as well as anti viral properties. Of the three types of interferon alpha and beta bind the same receptor and are more antiviral and less immunomodulatory. Gamma interferon is more immunomodulatory and less antiviral in its effect

The efficacy of interferon treatment is now well documented. Conversion from HBeAg to Anti e or HBsAg to Anti HBs is seen in 30-40 % and 10-15 % patients respectively however spontaneous seroconversion rates are around 10 and 2 percent respectively. Relapse to a replicative state i.e. from Anti HBe to HBeAg positive occurs in 10 to 20 percent of successfully treated patients but this usually occurs after one year. The accepted dose of interferon is 5 million units daily (MIU OD) or 10 MIU twice weekly for 16 wk. The treatment may need to be extended up to six months or further in some cases. Side effects of interferon use include fatigue headache, myalgia, nausea, vomiting, irritability, depression and hair loss. Marked neutropenia, thrombocytopenia and seizures may require temporary or permanent discontinuation of therapy. Retinopathy and autoimmune thyroiditis may be rarely seen.

Antiviral agents presently in use are nucleoside analogues. These are primarily Lamivudine and famcyclovir. Lamivudine inhibits the reverse transcriptase, which is necessary to transcribe HBV RNA pregenome to HBV DNA. The drug used in doses of 100 mg per day orally is effective in not only suppressing viral replication but also in converting from HBe antigen positive state to anti Hbe and also leads to improvement in the necroinflammatory scores on liver biopsy. This drug is discussed in detail elsewhere.

Lamivudine is a nucleoside analogue, which interferes with viral replication. Usually recommended in doses of 100 mg/day it causes an acute drop in the levels of viral DNA within days of administration. Lamivudine is recommended to be taken form between one to three years and a moderate degree of sero conversion from 'e' to anti-e state is widely reported. It has no serious side effects and can be prescribed in children as well.

Newer approaches to eradicate HBV infection.

Antisense approach involves the blocking of transcription and translation of DNA and RNA by antisense molecules or ribosymes that are complementary to the viral DNA or RNA. Adoptive immunity transfer was contemplated as a form of treatment when in one instance bone marrow transplant of Anti HBs positive and Anti HBc (IgG) positive donor led to clearance of HBsAg in a chronic HBV recipient. Hence it is possible that in vitro stimulation of autologous lymphocytes can lead to successful immune manipulation. Selective targeting of antivirals to the liver has been tried recently. Antivirals conjugated to ligands directly reach liver cells with heightened efficacy and a lower incidence of side effects. Presently lactosaminated albumin and recombinant chylomicrons are being tried as ligands for antiviral agents

Vaccines are a cheap and promising form of therapy, which would induce powerful humoral and cellular immune responses and viral clearance. S and Pre-S Antigen vaccines are being contemplated as agents, which may lead to viral clearance. DNA Vaccines using plasmid DNA which expresses viral proteins in situ can stimulate Anti HBs production and stimulate viral clearance in mice in presence of HBV infection as it stimulates a powerful B as well as T cell response. T-Cell vaccines, which use cytotoxic T cells primed with viral antigens, may induce viral clearance when injected in chronic HBV infection.

It is very likely that the ideal form of therapy evolved in future would be a combination of two or more of the modalities of treatment described above. It remains to be seen if these new approaches withstand the test of controlled human trials and subsequently actual clinical use.

Dr. Vinay K. Thorat
39/36, Erandwane, Prabhat Road, Lane 9B, Pune – 411 004
Tel : 5662035 (O), 5441080 (R) E-mail : vkthorat@vsnl.com

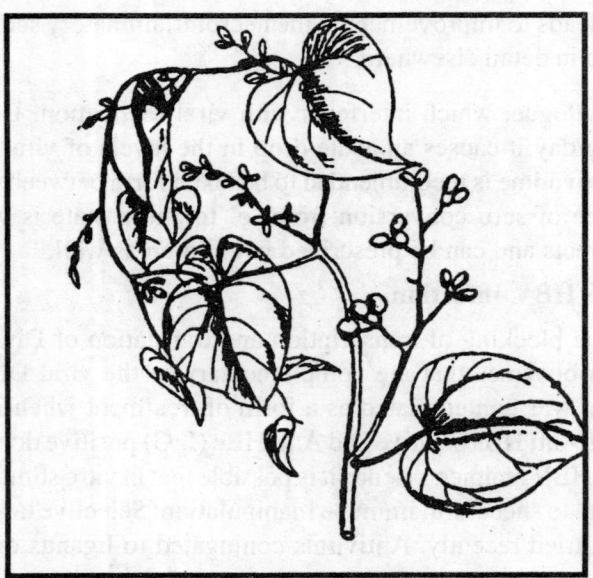

Sanskrit Name : Guduchi
Latin Name : Tinospora cordifolia

Hepatic Disorders

Clinical Interpretation Of LFT With Ayurvedic Point Of View.

Dr. Mali M. D.
Prof. Dr. Kulkarni P. H.

The liver is the central organ of metabolism in the body. Although it constitutes only 2% of total body weight, it receives 28% of cardiac output.

Hepatic activities are directly reflected in many of the substances circulating in the blood and are also present in other body fluids.

Although hepatic functions affect many metabolites, certain tests and manipulations correlate particularly well with the structural and functional integrity of the liver; these determinations are conventionally considered as liver function tests.

To gain an understanding of how these tests are to be interpreted from point of view of Ayurvedic samprapti and for Ayurvedic treatment view is the main goal of this article.

Most of the liver function tests provide quantitative information about broadly defined abnormalities and can not further discriminate the causes, however the patterns of abnormalities in several different liver function tests can be helpful in better delineating some hepatic disorders.

Because the liver has such substantial reserve capacity, hapatocellular loss must be a advanced before it becomes clinically apparent.

It is possible to detect on going hepatocellular damage by measuring functional indices and observing in the circulation the products of damaged or necrotic hepatocytes.

Hepatic Disorders

Normal Path way for Billirubin

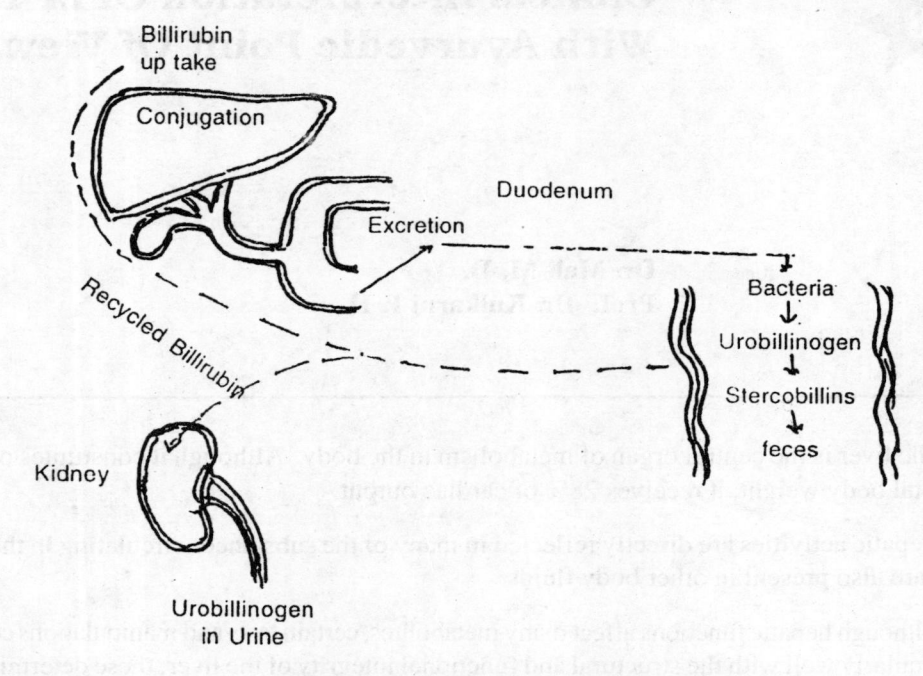

- Billirubin up take
- Conjugation
- Duodenum
- Excretion
- Recycled Billirubin
- Kidney
- Urobillinogen in Urine
- Bacteria ↓ Urobillinogen ↓ Stercobillins ↓ feces

Obstructed Path of Billirubin

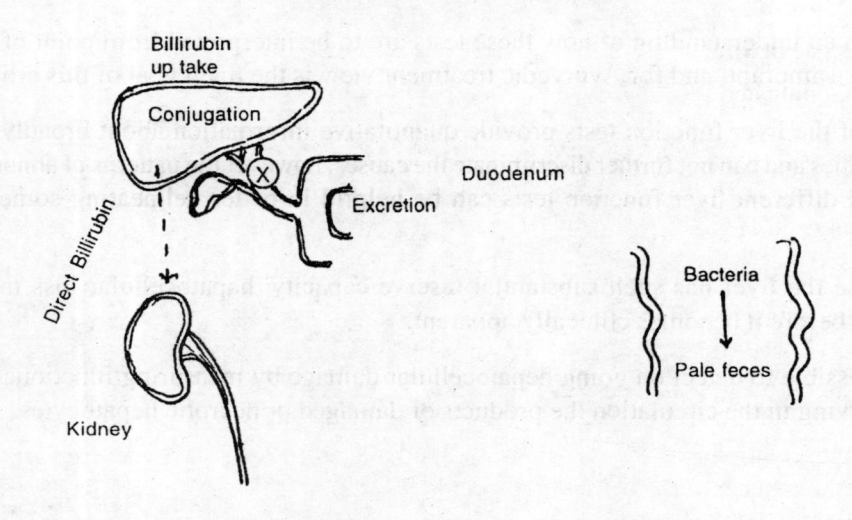

- Billirubin up take
- Conjugation
- X
- Duodenum
- Excretion
- Direct Billirubin
- Kidney
- Positive bile Urine
- Bacteria ↓ Pale feces

60

Hepatic Disorders

Billirubin Metabolism

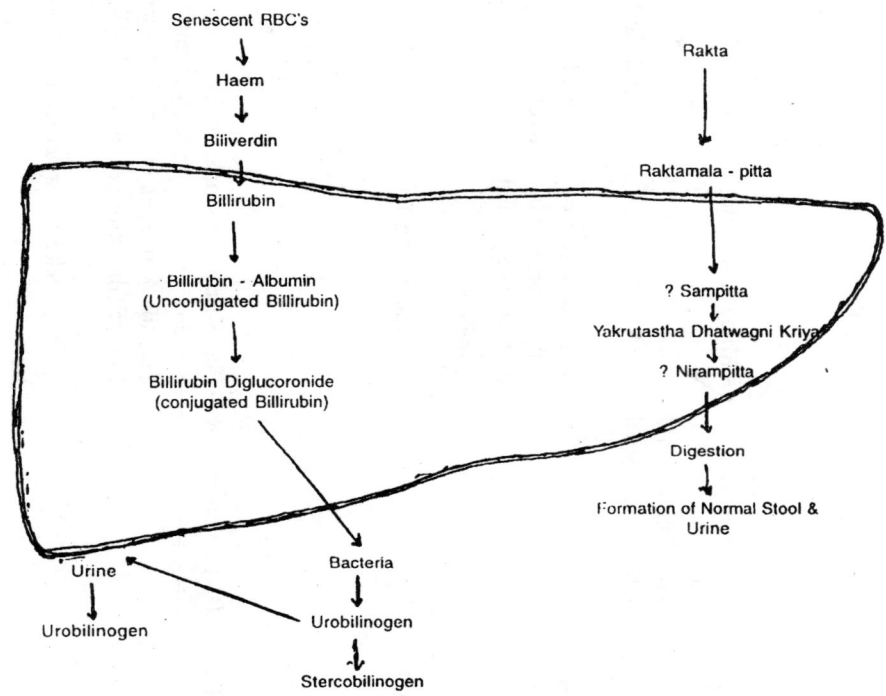

```
Senescent RBC's                              Rakta
     ↓                                         ↓
    Haem                                  Raktamala - pitta
     ↓                                         ↓
  Biliverdin                               ? Sampitta
     ↓                                         ↓
  Billirubin                         Yakrutastha Dhatwagni Kriya
     ↓                                         ↓
Billirubin - Albumin                      ? Nirampitta
(Unconjugated Billirubin)                      ↓
     ↓                                      Digestion
Billirubin Diglucoronide                       ↓
(conjugated Billirubin)              Formation of Normal Stool &
     ↓                                       Urine
  Urine        Bacteria
     ↓            ↓
Urobilinogen  Urobilinogen
                  ↓
            Stercobilinogen
```

Following pathophysiological events can be considered according to Ayurvedic views :

1) Increase in Sr. Bilirubin = Pittaviridhi - Ati pravruti
   - Conjugated Bilirubin = ? Niram Pitta
   - Unconjugated Bilirubin = ? Sam Pitta
2) Decreased Hepatic uptake ⎫ Yakruta Dhatwagni Mandya
   Decreased Hepatic conjugation ⎭ Saman Vikruti
3) Hepatocellular damage = Yakruta Shotha/Pak
4) Billiary stasis = Sang
5) Steostasis = Medomay Yakrut, Medoj Siragranthi
6) Cirrhosis = Yakrut Shosh

Tabular presentation of events related with liver, related LFT changes and its interpretation Shrotodushti Prakar, effect on Malamutra, and Treatment principle gives us detailed and minute pathophysiology and liver disease and samprati bhed by proper intrerpretetion and choice of drug.

Hepatic Disorders

Pathological event	Changes in LFT	Types of Shrotodushti	Effect on stool & Urine	Treatment Principle	Drug of choice
1. Prehepatic increased production of Bilirubin	Total Bilirubin increased	Pittavridhi	Mutrapitata	Pitta pachak, Shamak	Tikta Rasa Suvarna Suth Shekhar
	Uconjugated hyper Bilirubinaeamia Conjugated = Unconjugated	↑ Sampitta Ghruta Normal Yakrutdhatwagni Provocation of Pitta	Dark coloured stool	+ Mild Purification	Amalaki+ Kasis +
			Direct Bilirubin in Urine Dark coloured stool		Aryogya Vardhini
	Unconjugated hyper Bilirubina-eamia + ALP↑slightly	Provocation of Pitta → Stasis → obstruction → Vimargagaman	-"-	Removal of stasis without increase in its quantity e.g. mild purgation	Phalatrikadi Kadha
	= ↑ Unconjugated Bilirubinaeamia+ ↑ALT, ALP	Degeneration of Yakrut Dhatu	-"-	+ Invigorate the liver	
2. Hepato-cellular damage i) Acute	Sudden ↑ Bilirubin, ALT↑↑↑ AST ↑	Provocation of Pitta by Ushna & Tikshna → Yakruta pak	Dark colour stool & Urine	Pitta Shaman by Mrudu Praval, Snigdha	Su. Makshik
				Stop the Activation of liver cell digestion i.e. (Pak)	Amlaki, Godanti, Aroyga Vardhini.
				Mild to moderate purgation	Kharjuradhi Manth
				Invigorate the liver	Punarnavamandur.

62

Hepatic Disorders

Pathological event	Changes in LFT	Types of Shrotodushti	Effect on stool & Urine	Treatment Principle	Drug of choice
	Acute fall in ALT, AST ALP, Bilirubin without clinical improvement	Arishtasuchak i.e. Fatal Signs	"-"	"-"	Bad Prognosis.
ii) Chronic	Bilirubin levels rises slowly- ALT↑ AST↑ALP↑, Sr.proteins↓ - albumin ↓↓	Slowly Provocation of Pitta Degeneration of Yakrut dhatu, Stasis of Dosha, Yakrut Dhatwagni Mandya	"-"	Long duration of treatment - Invigorate the liver ↑Digestive power of liver. Purification of dosha for long duration.	Rejuvenating treatment alongwith above treatment.
3. Cholestasis i) Intra Hepatic (Medical jaundice)	Bilirubin↑↑, conjugated Bilirubin ↑↑↑ ALT↑↑,AST↑, ALP↑↑↑, Sr. Bilesalts↑, Proteins usually normal	Provocation of Pitta → Stasis → obstruction → vimargagaman	Dark Yellow coloured urine, stool pale or clay coloured	Normalisation of Saman vayu, pitta-shama, ↓ process of degeneration, relieve the obstruction without ↑ in quantity, moderate purgation.	Punarnavamandur, Punarnavakwath, KumariKalpa, Trivrita leham
ii) Extra Hepatic a) Partial	Fluctuating Sr.Bilirubin levels Conjugated Bill.↑↑ Sr.Bilesalts↑, ALP↑↑ ALT↑ AST↑ Sr. cholesterol ↑	obstruction →Stasis → vimargagaman	Dark coloured stool & Urine	Relive obstructions with or without ↑, in quantity of Pitta, Strong purgation → pittashaman, Invigorate the liver.	Tamrabhasma with lime juice Gorochan with Gomutra. Navayas loh. Trikatu

Hepatic Disorders

Pathological	Changes in LFT & Urine	Types of Shorotodushti	Effect on stool choice	Treatment Principle	Drug of event
b) Complete obstuction	Conjugated Hyper bilirubinamia, Bilesalts↑, ALP↑↑↑, ALT may raised Sr.Cholesterol ↑↑	obstruction → Stasis → vimargagaman	Clay coloured stool dark coloured urine.	No purgation still obstruction is relieved. Surgical intervention Medopachak, Ushna tikshna guna.	ArogyaVardhini TrikatuChurna
4. Cirrhosis	Sr. Bilirubin ↑↑ ALT ↑↑	Yakrut Shosh(Ruksha guna) →Saman Vayu	Dark coloured urine ↓ quantity	Snighdhaghrita, Invigorate the liver	Mahatiktakghrita, Maharohitak,
	A/G Ratio reversed	Stasis of Pitta ↓ of Raktadhatwagni Malformation of next dhatu.	Kled Nirmitee↓↓	Yakrut Samya Dravya Nityamev virechanam ! Yakrut Soup	Kalyanakghrita, Yakrut Soup
5. Fatty liver	Sr.Bilirubin↑↑ Sr. proteins ↑ ALT↑↑ Sr.Cholesterol ↑↑	Medomaya Yakrut Medoj siragranthi Stasis → vimargagaman	Avilpita mutrata Shrista, Alpapita malapravrutti	Medo pachak, Pittashamak Kapha Nashak Yakrut Ballya	Asavarishta Kalpana, Haritaki + Sharpunkha with honey TamraRohitak RohitakArishtam KutakiYavakshar Mandurvatak KumariAsav.

Hepatic Disorders

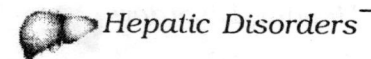

Choice of drug

Drugs Names listed in tabular presentation are not only the drug of choice but one can select the drug as it is by keeping the same principle of treatment.

Phaltrikadi kashay

Tikta rasa being Pittashamak and Rasraktapachak it could be beneficial in such sampittavirudhi.

It also works as rejuvenating drug for Raktavah Srotas.

Destruction of RBCs can be reduced by reducing ushnatwa and tikshnatwa of Pitta i.e. it reduces the pre hepatic excessive bilirubin production due to Haemolysis.

Amlaki + Kasis bhasma along with ghee

after proper treatment of haemolysis for pandunashan and being as rasayan. You can give the above mixture.

Acute hepatatocellular damage

Is due to increase Ushnatwa and Tikshnatwa leading to Yakrutpak.

It can be stopped by Madhur, Atisheet, Prawal pishti, Suvarna Makshik, Godanti, Amlaki. These drugs may reduce activation of liver cell damage by Pittashaman.

Arogya Vardhini

It is a rasayan drug. It invigorates the liver, It gives stimulation for proper bile secretion and excretion. It also works as a mild purgative due to Kutki.

Kharjuradi Mantha

It is Mahur, Snigdha, and Shita. It subsides the provoked pitta, reduces fatigue, thunder.

Punarnava Mandur

It is Tridosh shamak, Punarnava being anti inflammatory, it reduces the shotha of the liver cells. Mandur is Kashaya, Madhur Shita. It reduces Pitta and Kapha by Katu Vipak. Punarava Mandur work as cleaning the channels, increases digestive power of dhatu. It regulates the liver secretion and excretion.

Tamrabhasma alongwith Lime juice

It works as bhedana and shrotoshodhan, along with limejuice it also increases the secretory activity of glands like liver. It is useful in Bahudoshavastha.

Gorochana with Gomutra.

It is useful in partialy obstructive pathology. It increases the quantity of pitta and release the obstruction and it also enhances the flow of Pitta from shakha to KoshthaGhrita kalpana

The process of cirrhosis takes place due to rukshaguna of vata and Ushna, Tikshna guna of pitta due to excessive Katuahar kalpana. Gritakalpana stated in kamala pandurogadhikar

Hepatic Disorders

are Mahatiktak, kalyanak, etc. are good for cirrhotic liver.

Sharapunkha Haritaki with honey

Sharapunkha reduces the liver enlargement. It gives rejuvenation to hepatocytes. Haritaki and honey reduces the kleda and hence it is more useful in alcoholic liver diseases.

Kutki

Useful in conditions like biliary stasis in hepatocytes, fatty liver, partial obstructions due to gallstones.

It suppresses the Kapha and reduces the kleda due to Katu rasa, Ruksha and Ushna. It normalize the secretary and excretory activity of Hepatocytes.

Mild to moderate purgation?

Bile itself work as irritant for intestines. Strong purgatives can increase irritability of intestine leading to intestinal ulcer and other essential electrolytes also lost due to strong purgation. Strong purgation may increase the vatadosha therefore we must have to use the drugs, which are Madhur, Kashaya, snigdha e.g. Haritaki, Triphala, Gandharva haritki, kutki, Araghvadh.

Dr. Mali M. D. (M. D. Scholar)
A/p. Malgaon, Tal. Miraj, Dist. Sangli – 416 407
Tel : 0233 – 266522, 266717 Pune – 020 – 7291795

Hepatic Disorders

Introduction To Hepatitis 'C' And It's Ayurvedic Management

Vaidya Dhananjay J. Khajgiwale

Definition :

Hepatitis C is the inflammation of the liver due to hepatitis C virus. This can causes long-term complications and hence difficult to overcome. Mostly results in hepatic cirrhosis and then liver failure.

Mode of Transmission :

Mostly transmits through Blood transfusion, contaminated blood & blood products intravenous drug abuse, ear or body piercing tattooing needles. Dental procedures etc. sexual transmission is uncommon. Transmission from mother to foetus – 5% risk.

Tests for detection :

Enzyme immunoassay (EIA) which detect HCV antibodies with 95% surity. But it may give false +ve results. Confirmatory test is recombinant immunoblot assay (western Blot) i.e. highly sensitive polymerase chain reaction (PCR) amplification.

Symptoms :

Most people suffering from hepatitis C **do not show** symptoms. It is difficult to diagnose.

    20% show symptoms like fatigue, appetite loss, and muscle pain.

    25% show jaundice.

    Fatigue increases with chronicity.

Global incidence :

Total world – 3% people infected

    = 170 – 200 million people.

    -     9 million Europeans.

Hepatic Disorders

- 4.5 million Americans.
- 4 times more common than HIV.
- 1000 deaths annually in U.S.A.

Country	Population affected (millions)
China	50.8
Egypt	10.5
Vietnam	4.5
Japan	2.8
France	0.667
Spain	0.288
U.K.	0.25

Progression of the disease :

85% patients go in **fibrosis** out of which most go in cirrhosis.

Liver biopsy may be done.

Hepatocellular Carcinoma may be developed.

Genotypes :

It refers to the genetic make up to an organism. There are <u>at least 6 different</u> genotypes of HCV & 50 subtypes.

Treatment :

Only interferon – 20% success.

Interferon with ribacitin – 40% success.

Ayuvedic Treatment :

This may be considered as a case of Kamla & complications come under Udata

Following combination is useful :

N. Stellata seeds	250 mg.
Abhrak Bhasma	250 mg.
Pippali (Piper longum)	100 mg.
Pittapapda (Fummaria parviflora)	100 mg.
Guduchi (Tinospora corditolia)	100 mg.
Punarnava (Boerhaavia diffuso)	100 mg.

Hepatic Disorders

Amalaki (Phyllanthus emblica)   100 mg.

1000 mg. = 1 gm.

1 gm tds dose.

Explanation :

1. N. Stellata – seeds were tested against carbon tetrachloride CCl_4 induced hepatatoxicity in rats & mice. The extract at 300 mg. / kg. i. p. markedly reduced the prolongation of sleeping time & significantly prevented the CCl_4 increase in wt. Vol., of liver & mortality.

The extract also prevented the necrosis of liver tissue and promoted to some extent liver regeneration.

2. <u>Indicia Mangiteria :</u> has reported to show protection against CCl_4 induced liver injury by preventing liver cells.

3. <u>Pippli :</u> Used in ascites

4. <u>Pittapapda :</u> Used as liver tonic.

5. <u>Guduci :</u> Used as anti-inflammatory (liver) shodhan & liver tonic.

6. <u>Punarnava :</u> Used mainly in ascites.

7. <u>Amalami :</u> Used as Pittashamak.

8. <u>Abhrak Bhasma :</u> Used as tonic

Above combination is useful in Hep. C

Vaidya Dhananjay J. Khajgiwale B.A.M.S. Ph.D.
570, Narayan Peth, Nr. Kesari office, Pune 411 030. Ph. No. : 4452885 / 5460778

Hepatic Disorders

Hepatic Disorders And Imaging

Dr. Vilas A. Dole.

Introduction :

Up to about 40 to 50 years back x-ray films and Fluoroscopy i.e. screening were the only modalities available at our disposal by which actual images of various internal organs were obtained for diagnostic purpose. During last few decades due to mind-boggling advances in the science and technology, especially in physics and electronics there are many more modalities by which images of internal organs can be obtained. Ultrasonography and MRI are just a few to mention. Radiology, the name given to science of obtaining & interpreting X-ray images is better known presently as 'imaging science'.

Hepatic disorders including disorders of biliary tract happen to be a significant diagnostic problem for a general practitioner as well as a specialist. For proper and speedy diagnosis he has to depend upon various imaging investigations. For proper & just advice to the patient, the referring doctor must know exactly which imaging technique is to be advised for suspected hepatobiliary disorder.

In this article an attempt is made to enlist various imaging modalities available to us and indications of such investigations, in patients of hepatobiliary disorders.

For any suspected hepatobiliary disorder, the imaging modalities available are as under,

i) Conventional Radiography
ii) Ultrasound Scanning
iii) C.T. Scanning
iv) Radionuclide or isotope scanning
v) M. R. I. scanning

Hepatic Disorders

Conventional Radiology :

It includes the following procedures;
- a) Plain X-ray abdomen
- b) Oral Cholecystography
- c) I. V. Cholangiography
- d) Operative Cholangiography
- e) 'T' tube Cholangiography
- f) Percutanious transhepatic Cholangiography
- g) Endoscopic Retrograde Cholangiography

(a) Plain X-ray abdomen – this is a basic and very useful investigations for most of the hepatobiliary disorders. It rules out various types of gallstones, abnormal calcifications in the hepatic region, gives fairly correct idea about the size of liver. It also acts as a base line control film for other advanced imaging techniques.

(b) Oral cholecystography – Radio-opaque contrast medium, which concentrates in the gall bladder after 12 to 14 hours, is given to the patient per orum. Films exposed after this period shows gallbladder filled with contrast medium. Cystic duct is also visualized. This investigation gives fairly good idea about size, shape, and position of gallbladder. Function of the gallbladder can also be judged on this test. Nonradio-opaque calculi are visualized as filling defects, however if the gallbladder is functioning poorly this investigation is of little use.

(c) I. V. Cholangiography – This investigation is meant to visualize the bile duct. After a control plain film, contract is injected intravenously. After about twenty minutes it appears in the bile duct & then films are exposed in different planes. Tomographic techniques are many times required.

This investigation is becoming obsolete very fast because bile duct is usually investigated during cholecystectomy operation with operative Cholangiography.

(d) Operative Cholangiography – This investigation is carried out in the operation theatre. Many time pathology of gall bladder is associated with pathology of common bile duct also. Therefore, during cholecystectomy a small incision is made over cystic duct through which a small catheter is passed in to common bile duct. Sufficient amount of contract is injected while films are exposed. It rules out presence of stricture, stone or growth in common bile duct. As the contrast medium is directly injected in to the duct, it is also called as direct Cholangiography.

(e) T' tube Cholangiography – This is another 'Direct Cholangiography'. During operation

Hepatic Disorders

of cholestectomy a 'T' shaped tube is inserted, where one transverse arm of T is in the common bile duct and the other is in common hepatic duct. The long arm of T is kept outside the body. After about 7 to 10 days, a period generally required for Lysis of blood clots inside the ducts, contrast medium is injected & films are exposed so that the intraluminal abnormalities can be detected or can be ruled out.

(f) Pecutanious transhepatic Cholangiography – Significant number of patients do not get relief from pain for which cholecystectomy was performed. In such cases a small stone in the duct or stricture of the ducts are to be ruled out. To visualize these structures after cholecystectomy, a long needle is passed in to liver percutaniously under perfect aseptic precautions and under anesthesia. Contrast medium is slowly and continuously injected in sufficient quantity & concentration and then films are exposed in different planes so as to visualize required structures.

The main indications of this investigation are -

i) Jaundice – especially when, there is dilemma in labeling it as 'obstructive'

ii) Postcholecystectomy syndrome – where symptoms persist even after choeystectomy.

Prothrombine time of the patient must be checked & it should be well within normal limits before subjecting him to these investigations. Adequate antibiotic cover is also a must.

(g) Endoscopic retrograde cholangiopancreatography – This technique is rapidly replacing percutainious transhepatic Cholangiography. The indications are similar i.e. to confirm obstruction and post cholecystectomy syndrome. An added advantage for this procedure is it can be performed even though prothrombine time is rather high. This procedure is contra-indicated when access to the duct in 2nd part of duodenum is not possible due to pyloric stemosis, duodenal deformities or cases of gastrectomies.

A side viewing duo denoscope is introduced and through this a fine catheter is passed in to common bile duct. Contract is then injected & films are exposed in required planes and angles.

Ultrasound scanning:

This noninvasive and safe technique is fast replacing conventional radiology in hepatic disorders as an investigation of first choice. Many conditions like cysts, abscesses, neoplasm degenerative changes & metastatic deposits can be diagnosed to a fairly good extent at the hands of an experienced Radiologist. Gallstones and other intraluminar abnormalities of gall bladder can be detected. The only prerequisite for this is at least six hours fasting.

Computerized Tomography :

This technique is new rapidly establishing it self as a very valuable diagnostic tool in hepatic disorders. The tomographic technique in X-ray radiography is highly enhanced by using axial planes. The images created can be viewed on computer monitor. Because multiple planes are used to image internal organs this is also known as body section radiology.

Both diffused and localized abnormalities of liver, can be well demonstrated. It can be used with contrast aided enhancement when findings are nonspecific or equivocal. Malignant tumors-primary & secondary, focal nodular hyperplasia, haemangioma, cysts, abscess etc. can be diagnosed more confidently with the help of this investigation.

Isotope Scanning :

An intravenous injection containing labeled isotope (i.e. an atom of an element having same atomic weight but different atomic number and hence possessing property of radiation) is given to the patient. The drug soon gets concentrated in to the tissue having specific affinity towards the drug. The area of the organ is then scanned to monitor the radiation. Principle behind this technique is diseased portion of the tissue shows decrease or no radiation. Normal parameters for area and amount of radiation are set with which diseased portion can be compared. Images seen over monitor of scanner can be transferred on films. Focal areas of diminished radiation are diagnostic. This technique is most widely used to detect and estimate metastatic lesions.

M R I Scanning :

Magnetic resonance can produce images of gallbladder and biliary tract. But it offers no added advantage over more cheaper and conventional methods of imaging like ultrasound & X-Rays. Role of MRI in liver disorders is still being estimated.

Summary :

There are many methods of obtaining images of liver & biliary tract for diagnostic purpose. In this article I have just mentioned various imaging techniques. Principles & indications of these are also mentioned. A doctor, especially a general practitioner, must have a basic knowledge of various imaging techniques as he is constantly working as a liason between patient & specialist. Nature of each investigation differs from patient to patient. It is better that considering physical, mental & financial position of each patient a doctor should advice for investigations so as to get optimum information.

As I have mentioned in the beginning of this article, the sciences of Physics & electronic are progressing very fast & newer techniques are immerging. Positron emission tomographic imaging is one of them. But its exact role in hepatic disorders and mainly its availability in our country & its cost cannot yet be imagined.

Hepatic Disorders

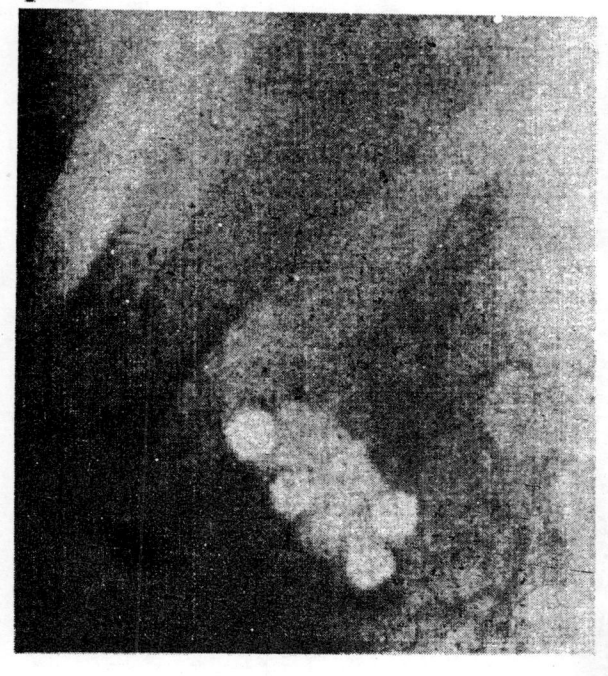

Plain X-ray abdomen showing Galstones

Oral cholecystography filled gallbladder & commonbile duct are seen

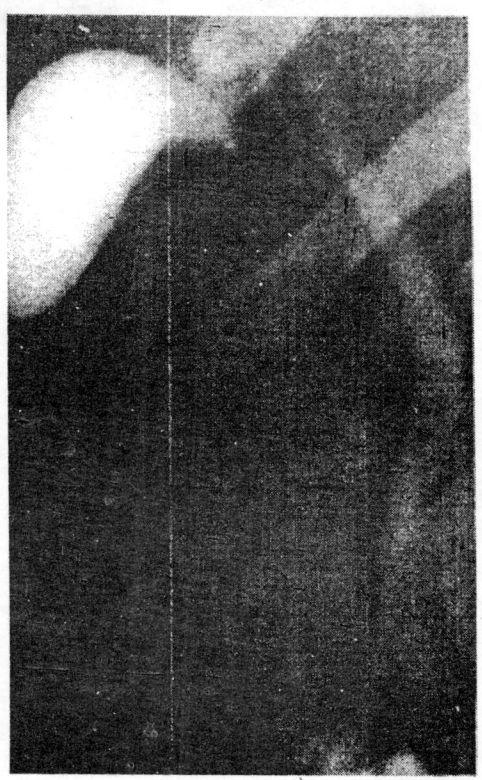

Hepatic Disorders

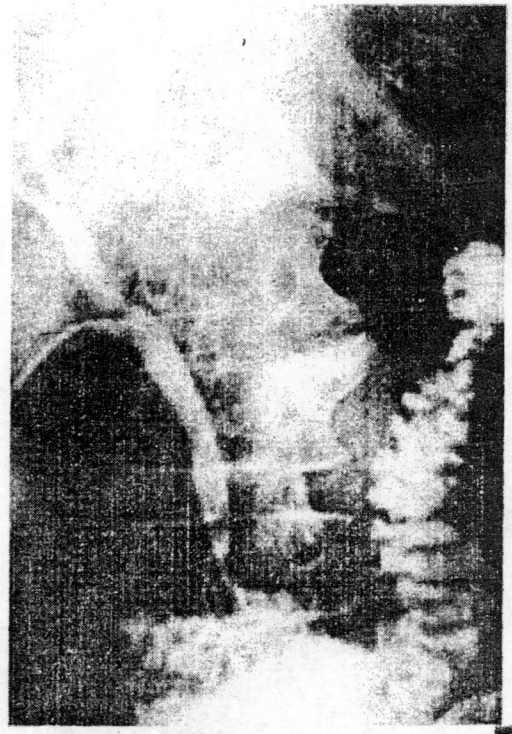

Operative cholangiogram small filling defect in the lower end of common bile duct due to stone.

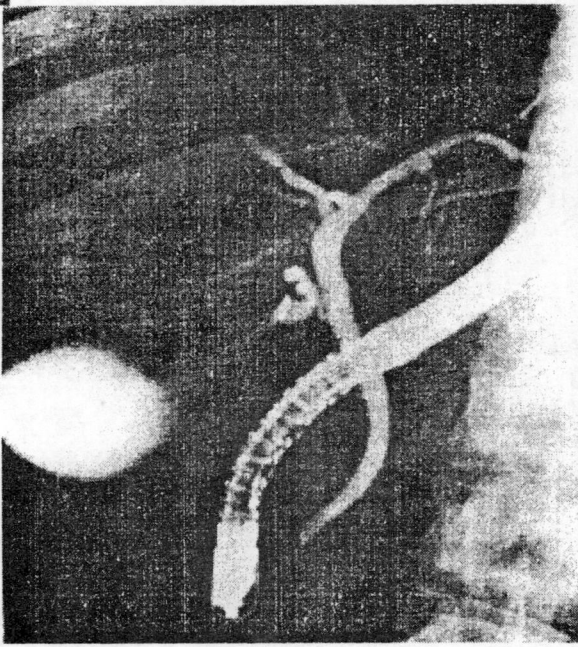

Retrograde cholangiography sideviewing due denoscope, common bile duct, hepatic can be seen

Hepatic Disorders

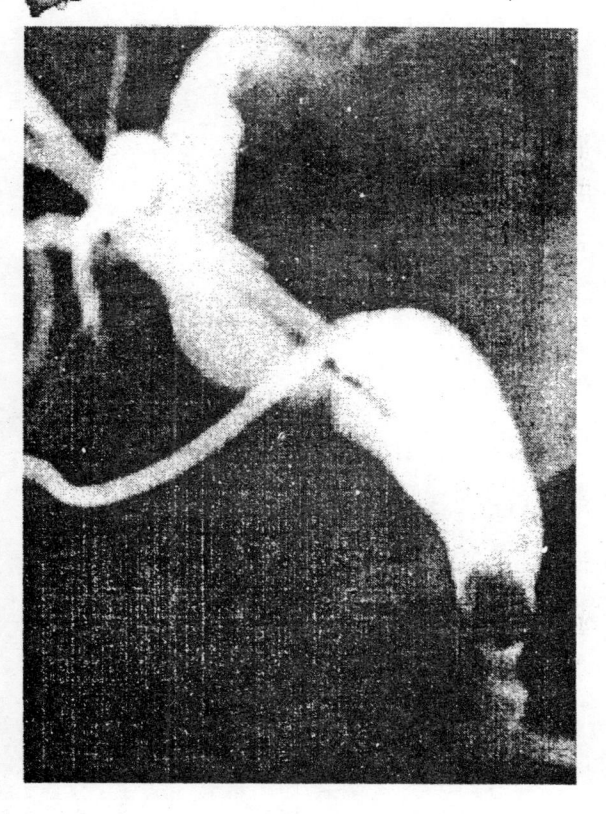

'T' tube cholangiography. Large filling defect in the lower end of common bile duct due to stone.

Dr. Vilas A. Dole.
Vice Principal & H.O.D. Radiology
T. A. M. V. & S.T.R.C.A. Hospital

Hepatic Disorders

Clinical Evalution Of Phalatrikadi Kwath And Arogyavardhini In Early Hepatic Cirrhosis : A Case Report

Wachasundar Nachiket
Wachasundar Neha

Abstract

A non-alcoholic, middle aged male patient was treated with

1. Arogyavardhini Ras 1gm. bid and 2. Phalatrikadi kwath 100ml. bid, for three months. The patient was relieved completely as far as the clinical and biochemical parameters were considered. However the ultrasonography reports showed no further increase in the hepatic cirrhosis.

Introduction

Hepatic cirrhosis is not a primary disease, but the end result of a diffuse liver injury secondary to poor nutrition, anoxia, action of toxins, alcoholism, various hepatic infections or biliary obstruction. There is a diffuse cellular necrosis that ends in a collapse, regeneration, fibrosis and altered hepatic circulation. A diffuse hepatic cell injury can also progress to a cirrhosis. So many acute lesions of the liver terminate as hepatic cirrhosis. The main abnormalities of a hepatic cirrhosis are;

1.Necrosis 2. Collapse 3. Regeneration 4. Fibrosis 5. Altered circulation.

A hepatic cirrhosis case may show following clinical manifestations :-

1. Loss of appetite
2. Hepatomegaly
3. Spleenomegaly
4. Ascites
5. Oedema of the legs

Hepatic Disorders

6. Fever
7. Diarrhea
8. Haematemesis
9. Jaundice
10. Portal hypertension
11. Anaemia

The case study

A 45 years old male patient visited our clinic four years ago. He was presenting all above clinical manifestations. He was having jaundice for last six months with no considerable effect in spite of a physician's constant, regular treatment. The patient was a vegetarian, non-smoker and non-alcoholic bank employee. He was not a tobacco chewier also. In his history he couldn't tell us any relevant relation to infectious disorder. No history of injections needle application or blood transfusion was noticed. His feaces were of normal colour. His jaundice was mild to moderate. He was severely anorexic. His liver was tender and slightly enlarged. His spleen was also tender and slightly enlarged. His gall bladder was not palpable. He was seeking antihyper tensive treatment for last three years.

Due to the limitations of the conventional medicines, he was referred to Ayurvedic physician by his consultant. The patient was then thoroughly examined clinically and advised to undergo biochemical as well as sonological examinations. The results of the said examinations are presented in the table.

The patient was then kept on strict Ayurvedic diet and treatment for further three months.

The diet comprised of cow's milk only 1 to 2.5 liters daily in three to four divided diet. All the rest of the foodstuffs along with water were strictly avoided. As the patient was obedient and co-operative he followed the dietary regimen scrupulously. Fresh cow's urine was also administered internally early in the morning on empty stomach. The dose was 30ml/day.

Besides the dietary regimen he was advised to take following medicines regularly;

1. Tab Arogyavardhini 1 gm. Bid with milk on empty stomach.

2. Phalatrikadi kwath (Ref. Sharangdhar Samhita : Madhya Khand kwath kalpana Prakaran)

Hepatic Disorders

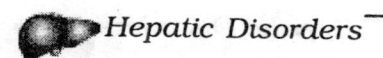

It contains following Ayurvediv medicines.

No	Ayurvedic Name	Botanical Name	Quantity	Part Used
1	Haritaki	Terminalia Chebula	2 parts.	Fruit pulp
2	Bibhitak	Terminalia belerica	2 parts.	Fruit pulp
3	Amalaki	Emblica officinalis	2 parts.	Fruit pulp
4	Amruta	Tinospora Cordifolia	1 parts.	Stem
5	Vasa	Adhatoda vasica	1 parts.	Leaves
6	Katuka	Picrorrhiza currora	2 parts.	Roots
7	Nimb	Azadiracta indica	2 parts.	Stem bark
8	Kirattikta	Swertia chirayata	2 parts.	Whole plant

Every day fresh kwath (Decoction) was prepared with using the above mentioned drugs.

Observations

The eleven main symptoms and signs mentioned above were considerably reduced in first fifteen days and were relieved completely in three months of period. Appetite was increased in first seven days. In the beginning he was consuming only 100ml. cow's milk. But after 3-4 days the quantity increased and after 15 days he consumed 1.5-liter cow's milk. His liver and spleen regained their normal size & shape. His jaundice disappeared. His blood pressure also turned to be normal. Ascites was considerably reduced.

Observation tables

I) Laboratory Investigations -

No.	Test	Before Treatment	After Treatment
1	Bile Salts in urine	+++	Nil
2	Bile pigments in urine	+++	Nil
3	Haemoglobin	8.56 gm%	13.86 gm%
4	ESR	64	6
5	Prothrombin Time	9.78	9.16
6	Serum Bilirubin		
	Total	12.36 mg/dl	0.62 mg/dl
	Direct	7.16 mg/dl	0.46 mg/dl
	Indirect	5.20 mg/dl	0.16 mg/dl

7	Serum Alkaline	404 Iu/l	103 Iu/l
8	Serum Total Proteins Phosphates	9.2 g/dl	7.39 g/dl
9	SGPT	269 Iu/l	32 Iu/l
10	SGOT	189 Iu/l	30 Iu/l
11	Australia Antigen Test HBS Ag.	- ve	- ve

II) **Ultrasonography**

No.	Particulars	Before Treatment	After Treatment
1	Liver size	Hepato megaly	Normal in size
2	Spleen size	Spleenomegaly	Normal in size
3	Ascites	Seen	Not seen
4	Hepatic cirrhosis	Seen	Seen

Conclusion

Thus from the above case study we can conclude that a case of hepatic cirrhosis can be treated successfully with Phalatrikadi kwath and Arogyavardhini. The said patient responded well to this treatment. However the cirrhotic changes in the lives are irreversible changes . the changes once happened can not be reversed but the hepatic functions can be maintained with the rest of the healthy hepatic tissue. Extensive clinical and biochemical study should be carried out to support this observation. But these cases can be improved with the said Ayurvedic treatment without any side effects.

This case is under my observation for last four years after completion of the treatment without any relapse.

Wachasundar Nachiket M. D. (Ayurved)
Wachasundar Neha B.A.M.S.
35, B/7 Mangalwar Peth, Karad 415 110 (M.S.)

Hepatic Disorders

How To Treat Hepatitis With Ayurvedic Methods

Dr.Dandekar Govind

The disease hepatitis is known since centuries. The word hepatitis means an inflammation of the liver, the largest gland in our body. It is differentiated according to the different causes of the disease. The type of hepatitis that I have dealt with in my book is the viral hepatitis, or a liver inflammation that is caused by viruses. The treatment of a disease depends on the etiology of the disease and its pathology. In case of the virus hepatitis the causative agent is a virus; but it is not a single virus. It is a group of viruses, and each of these viruses causes a different type of the disease. There was a lot of research on these viruses in recent years; and to understand the problem of viral hepatitis, it is necessary to know about this research. At present we know about six or seven different types of viruses, and each of them has a peculiarity of its own.

The longest known virus is the virus A. This virus is contacted through unhygienic conditions and is transmitted through foods and drinks. Virus A is very infectious! In India and other tropical countries it is quite common. The clinical picture is well known. In a few days after the infection the patient generally develops fever, pain in the limbs, gastrointestinal symptoms, and then the typical jaundice. The infection with virus A is seldom fatal and generally the patient recovers in a few weeks or even months. It is a disease that never becomes chronic. General supporting treatment is sufficient for the great majority of cases. The hepatitis E takes also a similar course, and no chronic cases are known. Hepatitis D is also not very important.

But its is a different story with hepatitis B and C. First the better known hepatitis B. The causative virus is generally transmitted through blood and blood products like globulin and plasma, infected injection needles, but also by sexual intercourse. This disease is known now for a few decades; but the hepatitis C is only known since 1989. Previously they used the term "non A-non-B-Hepatitis", because the blood tests showed that it was neither virus

Hepatic Disorders

A nor virus B; but it was no doubt-a virus hepatitis. This hepatitis is seldom acute. The signs and symptoms are uncharacteristic, jaundice is absent for the majority of cases. Only blood tests show that a liver inflammation and destruction of liver cells is going on. Further tests show that the virus is present in blood; and a liver biopsy shows that the liver is damaged. Usually this disease is also transmitted through blood products, transfusion and infected needles. But there must be other modes of transmission, as many times no cause can be found out. In Germany we have about 8,00,000 infected persons carrying the virus. In India it may be similar or even worse.

It is very important to know these different types of viral hepatitis, because the symptoms and prognosis are very different. Hepatitis A may recover spontaneously and is never chronic; hepatitis B becomes chronic in about 10% of cases, but hepatitis C becomes chronic in over 70% and may lead to cirrhosis of the liver and even to cancer of the liver. The modern medicine treats the hepatitis C with interferon alpha and Ribhavirin. Both are very costly and have many side effects. At present the chances of recovery are between 40% and 50%. How many will be cured in the long run is not jet known! A prophylactic vaccination against C is at present possible.

This was the situation as I considered the possibility of Ayurvedic treatment for this disease. In the modern medicine the treatment of an infection is to eliminate and to kill the causative organisms. That is how hepatitis C is being treated today, but the results are not very convincing. Can Ayurveda help ? The main difficulty is about the diagnosis. In the ayurvedic literature, there are references to two types of Kamala, Bahupitta kamala and rudhapatha kamala. The symptoms of bahupitta kamala can be compared with the viral hepatitis but there is no differentiation in the virus types and as you can very well imagine, one cannot compare the curse of hepatitis A with the cure of hepatitis C! It is also very difficult to diagnose hepatitis C with only clinical methods. Ayurveda has here another approach and another way of thinking. The primary cause of a disease is the derangement of the doshas and dhatus or dosha-dhatuvaishamya. The causes of this derangement are manifold. According to Sushrut there are seven different possible causes of a diseases. (You know them all). It is a common experience in an influenza epidemic that not every person, who comes into contact with the virus, gets it. It depends on the personal immunity of each individual. If we cannot kill the virus, then we must try to strengthen the resistance or the immunity of the patient. A patient who is having his dosha and dhatus in equilibrium will have a far better chance to cope with the infection than somebody who is not having this equilibrium.

In other words : we must try to increase the "health" of the patient. In this respect we have a lot of advice in Ayurveda. Only general instructions are not enough. We must give the instructions according to the constitution of the person. Ayurveda asks for a lot of modifications in the individual therapy. Every ayurvedic doctor knows that well-known Sutra-Deshan, Dushyam, palam, Kalam etc. I have tried to explain this with due modifications in

Hepatic Disorders

my book. The main difficulty for my treatment of hepatitis was, how to get the necessary medicines from India. A drug like Arogyavardhini was out of question! It is one of the important drugs in liver diseases, but anything that is containing even a small portion of mercury is prohibited here. If you give something like it here, you will be prosecuted. I could only use plants like phyllantus niruri, pricrorrhiza kurroa, Curcuma longa, Tinospora cordifolia and a few more. Another basic difficulty in treating hepatitis C with ayurvedic methods is the diagnosis. In the modern medicine the diagnosis depends on the pathological anatomy or the cellular pathology. We have not any such diagnostic methods in Ayurveda. Ayurvedic diagnosis depends on the symptoms and sings of the disease; and here again symptoms in an acute condition. The hepatitis C is essentially a chronic condition! Sometimes there are no symptoms, which give us a lead to the disease. Or they are not specific such as dyspepsia or fatigue. Sometimes hepatitis in the modern medicine is compared with the kamala in Ayurveda. Kamala does not mean jaundice! Kamala means tiredness, slackness! But in the description of the disease it is a predominant symptom! It seems that only the acute form the disease is known in Ayurveda but not the chronic form of hepatitis C! one cannot use the treatments used in India as there are no reports available about the specific treatment of hepatitis C!

I have tried to bridge over the gap between Ayurveda and modern medicine in my book, but it was not easy and it may be not acceptable for many ayurvedic physicians.

My main object was to show that with ayurvedic methods you can increase the health of the patient and put him into a better position (salutogenesis) to cope up with his illness and disease.

The hepatitis C is a good example for this type of treatment.

Dr. Govind Dandekar
Privatinstitut For Ayurveda, and Naturheil Kunde GbR, Halbinselstr, 43, 88142, Wasserburg

Hepatic Disorders

13. Standerdisation Of Certain Ayurvedic Drugs Used For Kamala

A. Saraswathy, S. Rukmani,
N. Meenakshi and R. Bhima Rao

Presently there is an increase in popularity of Ayurveda, which is clearly evident from the large number of people who are seeking advice the ayurvedic practitioners as they have no side effects and are low cost oriented. They have also been proved to be very useful in certain diseases such as peptic ulcer, asthma, viral hepatitis and diabetes, and in conditions, which are usually not curable, by modern system of medicine. The efficacy and growing popularity of herbal drugs have been endorsed by number of international organizations such as WHO, UNICEF and so on.

Standardization of these Ayurvedic medicines is an important task. Several factors influence the make-up of these herbal drugs as well as affect the batch to batch variability of the products' active ingredient. These factors include the actual herbal process. The only way to cure these that herbal drug preparations made with them, achieve optimum and consistent quality is to create and maintain a comprehensive quality assurance system that controls all steps of the manufacturing process. The active chemicals that are relevant to ensure efficacy and safety are to be used to characterise the quality of herbal drugs, besides analytical data. In the present study, three preparations viz. Chandra Prabha Vati, Navayasa Curna and Kalyanaka Guda described for KAMALA in the Ayurvedic Formulary Part-I were prepared in small scale with the authentic ingredients and final products were tested chemically. The evolved data will make it possible to established standards that can be used for the quality assessment for these drugs.

A. Saraswathy, S. Rukmani,
N. Meenakshi and R. Bhima Rao
Captain Srinivasa Murti Drug Research Institute for Ayurveda
Arumbakkam (CCRAS) Chennai 600 106.

Analysis Of Some Siddha Medicines Used For Kamala

A. Saraswathy*, M. Girija Rani and R. Sankari

Herbal therapy provides rational means for the treatment of many internal diseases, which are considered to be obstinate and incurable in other system of medicine. The traditional system of medicine viz. Ayurveda, siddha, unani, tibetan together with folklore systems continue to serve, a large portion of the population, particularly in rural areas, inspite to the advent of the modern medicines. The pharmacopoeias of these systems have mainly drawn upon the indigenous flora for the preparation of vide variety of herbal medicaments.

The Siddha Formulary of India – Part I mentions the use of 23 categories of herbal medicines including about 328 plant, which 13 compound drugs are described for the treatment of Mancal Kamalai / KAMALA (Jaundice). Talicatic Curanam, Venpucani Ilekiyam, Maka Elatik Kulikai and Kila Nellit Tailam were taken up for quality control in the standardization program of the Institute in lab. Scale and subjected to analysis. Thus the present paper deals with the chemical analysis and TLC / HPTLC profile of these hepatic protective potentials and the data presented will be useful in assessing the quality of these drugs.

A. Saraswathy*, M. Girija Rani and R. Sankari
Captain Srinivasa Murti Drug Research Institute for Ayurveda
Arumbakkam (CCRAS) Chennai 600 106.

Hepatic Disorders

Effect of Tamra Kumari In Liver Disorder

Vaidya Nikhil Kortikar.

Tamra is called more dangerous than poison still it is used in various drugs. Tamra's many preparations are used in Liver Disorders, one of it is Arogyavardhini.

Kumari i.e. Aloe vera is also used in Liver Disorders, and having very good results so if we write two good drugs together in different. Manner this is the main idea behind this project.

When I have started to find same old references at that time I came across the experiment of suvarnavacha by Vaidya P. Nanal. So, I rushed to Late Dr. Suitre to know about this project. So I have stated my Ph.D. work on this topic.

Preparation of Tamra Kumari

First of all we took baby plants of Aloevera from farm, & put them in small earthen pots full of sandy soil.

We selected 20 gauge copper wire's 5 cms. pieces for the projects. It was purchased from local shop. Then the classical purification process on all pieces was done.

Then we inserted copper wire in the stem of Aloevera and the plant was allowed to grow.

Observation of growing of Aloevera with copper. It was amazing that the tamrakumari was growing rapidly than normal.

Second noticeable thing was offshoots. The baby plant around Kumari were more in number. The size of each leaf was more & with more gel. After completion of 6 months we dissected the tamrakumari to see the state of copper wire & to my wonder it was totally absorbed.

That indicates the tamra was totally digested by plant. This is the another research project to find where that is assimilated. The project is going on.

Preparation of Drug of Tamarakumari

With the help of the some expert Vaidyas, We have prepared TK 2000. because of same restriction I will not explain the details of it.

Use of TK 2000 in Liver Disorders

30 pt of Kamala for the assessment of TK 2000 were observed.

We divided the group in two portion one will get the TK 2000 and other will get fresh plain Aloevera Gel in same calculated dose. Before starting the treatment we have done the LFT and after 10 days we again send the pt for LFT.

Out 15 pt's 12 pt got very good results.

3 pt got fair results in TK group and in other group 4 pt got good result. Rest of all got poor results.

Thus we can say that the drug prepared from tamrakumari is having good result than plain Aloe Vera.

Vaidya Nikhil Kortikar.
Ahemadnagar.

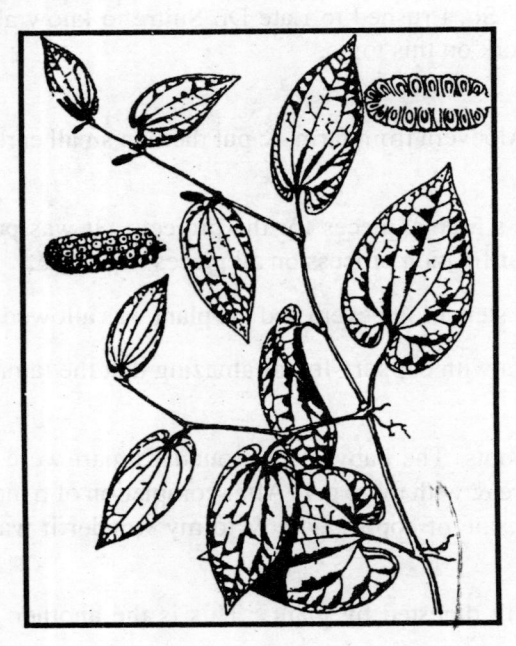

Sanskrit Name : Pippali
Latin Name : Piper longum

Hepatic Disorders

Prevention of Liver Disease

Dr. Deepak Amarapurkar.

Though exact prevalence of liver disease in India is not known, rough estimates can be made. Around 5% of the total hospital admission in our hospital which is 1000 beded tertiary care hospital are for the liver diseases and around 15% of patients admitted for other disorders are referred to the Hepatologist for various liver function abnormalities. Chronic hepatitis B infection is prevalent in 3 to 5% population in India suggesting that 45 million chronically HBV infected people are in our country and around 15 million of them suffer from chronic hepatitis / cirrhosis and or hepato cellular carcinoma. Similar data for hepatitis C; chronic infection 1 to 2%. 15 million infected people and around 3 to 5 million people suffer from chronic hepatitis / cirrhosis and / or hepatocellular carcinoma. In brief there is significant load of liver diseases on health care delivery system.

Viral hepatitis occurs mainly due to 5 types of viruses i.e. A, B, D, C, E. Out of these A & E are transmitted by feco-oral route (i.e. Enterically). Improving hygienic standards, supplying safe drinking water can prevent both these infections. In developed world where hygienic standards are good. Hepatitis A and Hepatitis E infections are practically non-existent. Current active vaccination for Hepatitis A is available which can give protective immunity against Hepatitis A. Currently Hepatitis E vaccine is being tested.

Hepatitis B, C, & D are parenterally transmitted and cause chronic infections. Paraenternal transmission can occur by infected needles, syringes, razors, toothbrushes, close contact with infected member, blood transfusion, sexual relation with infected members. Hepatitis B & C & D can be prevented by using disposable needles, syringes, razors and tooth brushes should not be shared. Hepatitis B vaccination programme when utilised in universal manner has been shown to have reduced Hepatitis B infection rates from 15 to 20% to less than 1% in countries like Taiwan & Thailand. Hepatitis D depends on B and hence prevention of Hepatitis B can automatically prevent hepatitis D. Hepatitis C infection is transmitted mainly

Hepatic Disorders

by blood transfusion and hence screening of blood for Hep C similar to Hep B and HIV should be done routinely. Unfortunately Hepatitis C vaccination is not yet available.

Other major cause of liver disease which accounts for almost 1/3 case of liver cirrhosis is alcohol abuse and hence reducing alcohol consumption or banning alcohol consumption can prevent significant burden of chronic liver disease. Judicious of drugs and early recognition of metabolic and inherited disease can also reduce the morbidity.

Much of the advice the physician gives patients relates to good general health priorities such as the need for a well balanced diet, regular exercise, and development of a comfortable ongoing relationship with a trusted physician. Much of this is just good common sense. Watching what one consumes and being aware of the special risks of travel to some parts of the world also makes sense. Then there are liver specific issues. Drinking in moderation means an occasional drink with no more than two drinks a day for a more and even less for a female. Avoiding the major risk factors that might lead to acquisition of viral hepatitis may require considerable changes in habits and hobbies. Relying on herbal medications or other alternative therapies as first line treatment of self diagnosed conditions may interfere with the patient receiving the correct effective medication. The patient needs to be aware of the occasional hepatic risks of any therapeutic medication with special attention to the potential for alcohol acetaminophen interactions, which may lead to liver injury. Vitamins in moderation seem safe however there is a risk of excessive vitamin A promoting further injury if liver disease is present.

Dr. Deepak Amarapurkar.
Consultant Gastroententerologist Bomabay Hospital
& Medical Research Centre, Mumbai.

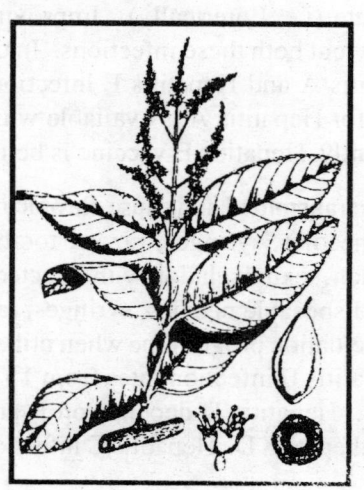

Sanskrit Name : Haritaki
Latin Name : Terminali chebula

Hepatic Disorders

Liver Diseases & Homoeopathy

Dr. Hari Gholap.

If someone asks, " How long you will live."

The answer is, "it depends upon his liver."

It proves the importance of liver.

Liver is important singular organ in the human body and does so many important chemical activities. In real sense, liver is chemical factory of human body. These chemical activities are essential for body physiology, which maintain the health.

Medical research is going on liver diseases all over the world but the common people are not aware of it. So, I decided to work on the topic **"Liver diseases and homoeopathy."**

Most of the liver troubles are due to bad food and drug habits. This starts from intrauterine life. This includes even so called safe drugs that pregnant woman takes. If this is toxic to mother's liver, are they not toxic to a foetu's liver? And later on, many babies are fed on bottle-feeding. Extra milk powder to the feed upset GIT and kidney and cause strain on the baby's liver. Such a baby is fretful, windy and colicky, suffers from constipation / diarrhea. Such a baby needs diluted feed to reduce the strain on liver. During the journey of childhood to adult and later on life, many food preservatives and artificial flavours are consumed in the food, which are hepatotoxic. Eating sausages, instant whip damages the liver. Consuming vitamins, iron, tonics for long time are harmful to the liver. Use of antibiotics, analgesics, tranquilizers, sleeping pills, stimulants, steroids etc. derange the liver. Drinking alcohol for long time, eating excess butter, cream, cheese, chocolates, coffee, eggs, fat & fried food deteriote the liver functions. Also eating excessive sugar, sedentary life, lack of exercise, constant stress & tension increase the liver complaints.

Medical science pays importance to the liver pathology but does not consider the liver when it is mearely under strain and in sluggish stage. Visible pathological changes occur later.

Hepatic Disorders

Now a days, we see many patients of liver disease. In my project, I selected patients from different groups such as age, sex, occupation, etc. Majority of the patients were suffering from yellow tinged urine, yellow eyes, loss of appetite, wt. loss, indigestion, flatulence, ascitis, weakness, etc. Fifteen main complaints were recorded. These patients were given the medicines as and when required, called for follow-up and observed for two years. Total number of patients selected were 156. Out of 156 pts. Majority were of infective hepatitis 110 (70.51%). The most effective medicines in this project were as follows.

a) Infective hepatitis 110 pts (70.51%) - Nux vomica 35 pts (31.81%)
Chelidonium 29 pts (26.4%)
Nat. Sulph 26 pts (23.7%)
China 21 pts (19.1%)
Sepia, lycopodium used.

b) Cirrhosis 23 pts (14.74%) - Nux. Vomica 8 pts (34.8%)
Chelidoxium 7 pts (30.4%)
Sulphur 8 pts (34.8%)
Lycopodium 8 pts (34.8%)
Phosphorus 8 pts (34.8%)
Nat. Sulph 6 pts (26.1%)

c) Obstructive jaundice 11 pts (7.05) - Phosphorus 4 pts (36.4%)
Nat sulph 3 pts (27.3%)
Podophyllum 3 pts (27.3%)
Hydrastis 4 pts (36%)

d) Haemolytic jaundice - Lachesis 4 pts (40%)
Calc. Carb. 2 pts (20%)
Mag. Mur 2 pts (20%)
Sulphur 2 pts (20%)

Other disorders of liver were given the indicated remedies.

In this project, 93 pts (59.62%) were cured, 17 pts (10.90%) were relieved, 21 pts (13.46%) did not turn up for follow-up and 4 pts (2.56%) were complicated.

While treating the patients of liver disease, their complaints, modalities, causative factors, constitution, desires & aversions, mental state, past & family history, investigations, susceptibility of the patient, etc. were considered.

In our project, nux-vomica, phosphorus, lycopodium, sepia, natrum sulph, china, lachesis, chelidonium, sulphur are found more effective in the liver diseases.

Following care should be taken during treatment of liver disease

Liver transplantation is physically not phisible and economically not viable. Following

Hepatic Disorders

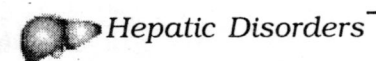

measures are useful during management of liver disorders.

1) Pt. should be under observation and should be given homoeopathic drugs as per indications.

2) Complete bed rest for about 1 to 1-5 months and then gradually increase the activities. But certain illnesses require longer rest.

3) Administration of minimum medications because most of the drugs are metabolised in the liver and few drugs are hepatotoxic and cause damage to the liver.

4) Diet – more calories – ample amount of fresh fruits, leafy vegetables, wheat, jawar, bajari, rice, nachani, pulses should be taken. Ghee, butter, oil should be minimum. Fat free cow's milk about ½ liter daily and buttermilk. Non-veg should be restricted. Minimum oil, spices and chilies. Patient can take daily one boiled egg.

5) For alcoholic liver disorder – abstinence from alcohol for at least 6 months to 1 yr. and observe the results. Ascitis pt should avoid-salt, baking powder and soda, tined food, salty food.

6) Vit. A, B, C, D & calcium should be given as per need.

7) When pt. Improves – mild exercise should be given and then gradually increase.

Prevention of liver diseases

1) Proper disposal of liver patient's excreta, urine, syringes, needles etc.

2) Consume boiled water.

3) Liver pt. should avoid – blood donations.

4) In the laboratory – no touch technique should be observed.

5) Use of disinfectant.

6) Vaccination – hepatitis – B vaccine should be given to the healthy individuals.

7) Avoid hepatotoxic drugs like Halothen, oral contraceptives etc. sleeping pills, stimulants, analgesics, excess paraceturnal, steroids etc.

8) Avoid – alcohol, charas, ganja, opium, tobacco, gutakha, cigarette, bidi, etc.

9) No sexual contact with hepatitis B + ve patients.

10) Moderate daily exercise in open dir.

11) Daily 10-20 minutes meditation.

12) Genus epidemicus in liver epidemic disease.

Dr. Hari Gholap
Amar Clinic, 135, Narayan Peth, Sitafal Baug, Pune – 411 030 (India)
Tel. : +91 – 020 – 4491974   +91 – 020 – 4472231

Hepatic Disorders

Awareness Of Hepatotoxicity And Protectivity.

Dr. Lalitha B. R. Ph.D.

Abstract

Hepatic disorders are difficult to cure, so awareness of hepatotoxicity and hepato protectivity is essential along with line of management in yakrit rogas. A travail is putforth to know about Hepatotoxicity, Hepatotoxic plants and Hepato-protective plants.

चिरञ्चरं प्लीहगदं यकृत रोगं सुदुस्तरम् ।

अग्रमासं तथा शोथं कांस्यकोडं सुदुर्जयम् ॥ रसेंद्र.सारा.संग्रह

Pathophysiology

Liver is the lever of life. It has many metabolic roles, it also immense capacity for self-repair, majority of the liver lesions observed in liver reverse rapidly on cessation of treatment. Repeated liver damage, failure can lead to liver cirrhosis.

Experimentally proved Hepato Protective plants

1.	Kalamegha	-	Andrographics panniculata	-	leaf
2.	Punarnava	-	Boerhavia diffusa	-	root
3.	Kasani	-	Chichorium inty bus	-	seed
4.	Eranda	-	Ricinus commuruis	-	leaves
5.	Saptarangi	-	Caseria esculenta	-	root
6.	Sharapunkha	-	Tephrosia purpurea	-	leaf
7.	Eclipta alba	-	Bhringaraja	-	leaves
8.	Nirgundi	-	Vigtex nigundo	-	Seed and leaves

Hepatic Disorders

9.	Guduchi	-	Tinospora cordifolia	-	stem
10.	Kakamachi	-	Solanum nigrum	-	whole plant
11.	Adhaki	-	Cajanuscajan	-	leaf
12.	Pippali	-	Piper longum	-	fruit
13.	Amalaki	-	Emblica officianalis	-	fruit
14.	Nimbha	-	Azadirachta indica	-	bark
15.	Daraharidhra	-	Coccinum fenestratum	-	leaf
16.	Bimbi	-	Coccinio indica	-	leaf
17.	Patola	-	Trichoranthus arbortristis	-	plant
18.	Parijata	-	Nycanthus arbortristis	-	leaf
19.	Ashwagandha	-	withania somnifera	-	root
20.	Sapota Parna	-	Alstonia scholaris		
21.	Maha Bala	-	Sidha rombhifolia		
22.	Ramphal	-	Anona muricata		
23.	Khadira	-	Acacia catechu		
24.	*Kadu garage	-	Fumaria parviflora	-	plant
			(in Hepatitis B)		
25.	*Picrorhiza Kurrao	-	Katuki (in Alcohol induced liver diseases)	-	root

26. Achyranthes aspera
27. Mangifera indica-bark
28. Garcinia kola, kolaveron
29. Tridex-procumbers-aerial part
30. Dianthus superbus
31. Schizandra chinensis
32. Butea monosperma
33. Aster canthus longfolia
34. Wedelia chinensis
35. Thujopsisdolabrata leaves (folklorein Japan)
36. Peumus boldus
37. Gymnosporia antisypilitica

Hepatic Disorders

38. Euphoria antisyphillitica
39. Aphamixus polystachya (rohitaka)
40. Silimarin from silibum maria (flavanolignins)
41. Withania frutecens
42. Rapharins sativus (mulaka)
43. Dacus carota
44. Glycerhizaglabra
45. Phylanthes amarus
46. Trianthema Postulacastrum

Hepato toxic plants

1. Gossy pium indicum
2. Terminalia oblongata-yellowood
3. Betavalgaris – beet pulp
4. Echium plantagium
5. Scnecio jacobaea
6. Helio tro pium eropeam
7. Crotolaria verrucosa
8. Lantana camera
9. Pyrrolizidine alka loids – derivatives
10. Cycadales
11. Lippia rehmanni
12. Myoporaceae (plants)
13. Ulmaceae (plants)
14. Casia auriculata
15. Atractylodes japonica
16. gentiana scabra
17. plantogo asiatica
18. citrus auranticum
19. polygonatum Japonicum
20. cyperus rotundus

Dr. B. R. Lalitha
No. 41, Chickanna Cottages, Loop lane of Race Course Road,
Bangalore – 560 009 Tel : 080 – 2254243

Hepatic Disorders

Panchakarma Approach To Physio-pathological Problems Of Hepatitis (Yakritdalyodar)

Prof. Dr. T. Srinivas Rao.

Yakritdalyodara of Hepatitis is a condition that disturbs and destroys the structural and functional normalcy of liver by DALAN and BHEDAN.

Inflammation, Necrosis and Cirrhosis of liver is caused by deranged DOSHAS. In this disease destroying the cell function, since the function of liver is the detoxification from toxins, chemicals and anti-biotics, the Hepatic cells bear the brunt, most

यकृद्दालयति दोषैर्भेयतीति यकृद्दाल्युदरम् ।

Physiologically liver, the largest organ in the body, consists of Kupffer cells, formed of endothelial phagocytic cells of reticulo endothelial system. The cells are so designed as to combat the complex function of more or less a powerhouse to perform as a full-fledged bio-chemical laboratory with maximum metabolic activity resulting in heat production sufficient for maintenance of a body temperature.

The cells are parenchymatatous, binucleated, polygonal with mitochondria and Golgi apparatus. The complex structure of liver cells is to perform diverse and complicated functions of secretion, oxidation, esterification, synthesis, metabolic deamination transamination and conjugation etc., speak of the intricate mechanism and reserve capacity of the liver and its remarkable quality of regeneration. Ayurveda consider liver as the seat of blood.

शोणित वहानां स्रोतसां यकृत् मूलं ॥ च ॥

The hepatic and portal circulation carries about 0.5 liters of blood per minute with varying degree of oxygen saturation from 80 to 100%. Liver at a given time can accommodate blood 1/3rd of the total volume of the body. Liver in Ayurveda true to its functions mentioned above is named as Yakrit.

यथा तथं करोतीते यकृतः ॥

Hepatic Disorders

meaning to bring back to normalcy the body tissues that are damaged and restores the body to its physiological state. In short liver is an organ that corrects the body abnormality and restores back the body to its normal state.

Pathology
Yakrit dalan in hepatitis

Hepato-cellular failure, nitrogen metabolism disturbances, leading to inflammation and necrosis of liver takes place in the liver substance due to viral infection from Hepatitis-A, Hepatitis-B, Hepatitis-C, Hepatitis-D, Hepatitis-E, Non - A and Non –B, due to which destruction of paranchymal cells to the DNA level, results in liver cirrhosis etc., leading to the obstruction of bile-canaliculi.

The above conditions resulting in reverse passage of bile into blood through hepatic vein and lymphatics, due to which serum bilirubin level rise above 2 mg % is sufficient to be termed clinically as JAUNDICE.

हरिद्र नेत्रः स मृशं हरिद्रत्वङ् नरवानन: ।
रक्तपीत शकृन्मूत्रो भेकवर्णो हतेन्द्रिय: ॥

Besides several other cause for increase in serum bilirubin level. i) In Gilbert's syndrome due to either to inability of unconjugated bilirubin to enter liver cells. ii) Disturbed hepatic function due to liver cell necrosis in viral hepatitis. iii) Inability on the part of hepatic cells to excrete conjugated bile through biliary canliculi, through some defect in hepatic excretory system called as Dubin Johnson Syndrome, the Rotar Syndrome. iv) Blockade of biliary flow through intrahepatic obstruction to the bile conaliculi or bile ductules cause extra hepatic obstruction of the bile duct.

All the above conditions are summed up in to two :

1. Obstruction at cellular level or bile canaliculi or Bile Ductules and at Bile duct level.
2. Defective hepatic function due to liver cell necrosis.

Samprapti

The blood due to excessive vitiation of "PITTA DOSHA" and further due to intake of Hot foods leads to the vitiation of PITTA.

तस्य पित्तमसृङ्मांसं दग्ध्वा रोगाय कल्पते ॥

Charaka has described the following types

कामला बहुपित्तेषा कोष्ठ शाखाश्रया मता ।
कालान्तरात् खरीभूता कृच्छ्रास्यात् कुम्भ कामला ।
कृष्णपीत शकृन्मूत्रो भृशं शूनश्च मानव: ॥ च.चि.

Hepatic Disorders

1. Koshtashrita kamala
2. Shakhashrita kamala
3. Haleemaka & kumbh kamamla

The primary lesion in icterus lies in the inflammed liver and the inflamed mucous of duodenum and its surroundings gastro-intestinal tract (KOSHTASHRITA) later on due to functional obstruction of liver. It takes bile to the abnormal levels of 5.2 kg. % and bile salt enters the Shakhas i.e. the DOSHAS migrate to SHAKHA from KOSHTAS. Thus concept of Ayurveda of SHAKHA and KOSHTSHRITA stands verified and proved.

Pancha karma approach

The pathology of KAMALA is said to be DOSHAS traversing to the SHAKHAS from KOSHTHA. They needs to be brought back in to the KOSHTA, by removing biliary tract blockade.

वृध्दया विष्यन्दनात् पाकात् स्रोतोमुख विशोधनात् ।

शाखां मुक्त्वामलाः यान्ति वायोश्च निग्रहात् ॥

For SHODHANA approach of PANCHAKARMA, of course preceded by SNEHANA along with liver corrective therapy is to be administered.

1. Daily doze of purgatives
2. Chologogue drugs like kutki
3. Medicated Ghees have to be administered

Samprapti vighatana – line of treatment

संशोध्यो मृदुभिरसकृत्तिक्तैः कामली तु विरेचनैः ॥

This line of treatment strikes at the root of the disease process by destroying and neutralising the inflammation and removes the obstruction and bring the DOSHAS, that have mis-adventured on to SHAKHA to its original seat of KOSHTA.

रेचनं कामलार्तस्य स्निग्धस्यादौ प्रयोजयेत् ।

पंचगव्यं महातिक्तं कल्याणकमथापि वा ।

स्नेहनार्थं घृतं दद्यात् कामला पाण्डु रोगिणे ।

Most physicians fear to adopt Ghrita treatment in Hepatitis due to fear of its non-digestion by duodenum due to absence of bile, but it has been proved by physiological experimentation that fat stimulates contraction of gall bladder and helps opening of sphincter of Oddi that guards the bile from entering into duodena. This may be clear by following lines from textbook of physiology.

Hepatic Disorders

(i) "Fatty foods, particularly creams, egg, yolk etc, are most effective stimulants, protein also stimulates to less extent, these factors cause contraction even when gall bladder is completely denervated." (Ref. Physiology by : C. C. Chaterjee)

(ii) "animal experiments have shown that high fat, low protein diet produces fatty liver. This observation has led to the false assumption that fats should be prohibited in viral hepatitis. Further more fatty changes in liver biopsy are never due to viral Hepatitis and if present are due to previous malnutrition. It is therefore a mistake to believe that fat is harmful in viral Hepatitis." (Ref. Text book of Medicine by S. K. Dutta)

Clinical trials on 60 patients in our hospital were recorded. The patients with viral Hepatitis were selected with higher serum bilirubin level. Encouraging results were noted with serum bilirubin returning normal after panchakarma and all the clinical symptoms of jaundice disappearing in 4 to 6 weeks.

Sr. No	Sex	No. of Patient Treated	Cured	Relieved	Otherwise
1.	Male	24	16	4	4
2.	Female	20	12	3	5
3.	Male child	8	5	3	-
4.	Female child	8	6	2	-

Line of treatment

1.	Pancha Gavyam Ghritam	5 Grams BD in the morning with milk
2.	Katuka Rohini	Fried 1 Gram daily in the morning
3.	Bhumi Amla Swarasa	50 ML one daily
4.	Katu Tumbi JAL	For Nasya Karma (Nasal Infiltration)
5.	Netranjan	Jyotishmati Swarasa

Further research trials in panchakarma line of treatment should be continued in Hepatitis, which is eluding the modern scientific advancement to find a definate cure in Ayurveda. Panchakarma speciality may bring a ray of hope towards cure of this disease.

Dr. T. Shriniwas Rao
Dierctor, S. H. E. S. Ayurved Hospital, Medical College & Research,
Gulbarga, Karnataka – 585 101 Tel. : 08472 – 25376, 25377

Hepatic Disorders

Clinical Assessment Of Shankhabhasma Vati (Rasashala) + Laghusutshekhar Vati & Indrayav Vati In Amoebic Hepatitis

Vaidya P. C. Yawatkar

Introduction

Amoebic hepatitis is diffuse, acute or chronic inflammatory disorder of liver caused by Entamoeba histolytica. It is clinically characterized by vague symptoms of long duration, associated with an enlarged and tender liver.

Amoebic hepatitis is an annoying and disabling disease, which reduces the working efficiency of an individual. It is definitely a challenging problem.

This paper presents a retrospective analysis of 40 cases from out patient department.

Materials and Methods

Hepatic amoebiosis is a common complication of the bowel infection. There is vagueness and variability of the symptoms in amoebic hepatitis. The patients included in this study were having stool test positive for Entamoeba histolytica, though negative fecal results do not exclude hepatic amoebiosis. Necessary and pertinent investigations were carried out to exclude the suspected cases of Liver abscess. Patients were selected at random irrespective of Sex, Caste, Occupation. Patients below age 15 years were not included in this study as the doses of medicines given were different.

All 40 patients were treated with 1) Shankhabhasma vati (Rasashala)

>> Dose-250 mg thrice a day with water.

> 2) Laghusutshekhar vati-

>> Dose-250mg thrice a day with water.

> 3) Indrayav vati-

Dose - 250 mg. thrice a day with water.

Ingestion Time - after Food.

Though the period of treatment given was different for every patient, the observations given in this paper are made after completion of 15 days treatment.

Observations

1) Highest incidence was noted in the age group of 21 to 30 years, followed by the group 31 to 40 yrs.
2) Male to Female ratio was 2 : 1
3) Peak incidence was Varsha Rutu, While lowest was in the Rutu Hemant.
4) Vatpitta prakruti patients were more in number, while incidence was noted low in Kaphapitta type.
5) Students were affected more, followed by servicemen.
6) Out of 40 patients
   a) 40 were positive for E. H.
   b) 40 were having pain in abdomen.
   c) 32 were having fever
   d) All the 40 patient had positive percussion test for tender liver.

As these 4 were main features / findings, effect of treatment on these four was observed to decide the results.

Results : Following Table shows effect of treatment after 7 and 15 days.

Sr.No.	Findings	No. of patients	
		After 7 days	After 15 days
1.	Negative stool test for E. histolytica	7	19
2.	Reduction of pain in abdomen	23	11
3.	Reduction in fever	14	10
4.	Negative percussion test for tender liver.	14	16

It shows that after 15 days treatment-

1) 65% patients showed negative stool report for E. histolytica.

2) 85% patients showed reduction in abdominal pain.

Hepatic Disorders

3) 75% patients became free from fever.

4) 75% patients became free from liver tenderness.

Discussion

Shankha bhasma is ushna, laghu, ruksha and teekshna. It is also described as Grahanirognashan. It acts as deepan and paachan and is proved to be beneficial in liver and spleen diseases.

Laghusutshekhar vati

This is useful in condition like saam-pitta. Ultimately it is benificial in dushti of ras-dhatu, which gives rise to (jwar) fever.

Indrayav is tridoshaghna, Sangrahi, katu. It acts as deepan, shoolnashak, jwarnashak, atisarnashak and krumighna. These properties are very benificial in amoebic hepatitis.

Chitrak is Katu, deepan, paachan, laghu, ruksha. It is also shophanashak, krumighna and shoolnashak. It is proved to be beneficial in liver diseases.

Conclusion

Combination of Shankhabhasma vati(Rasashala), Laghusutshekhar and Indrayav vati is proved to be very effective in Amoebic hepatitis.

Vaidya P. C. Yawatkar (M.D.)
I Floor, Chandralok Apt. Delhi Gate, Ahmednagar, M. S.(India)-414001.

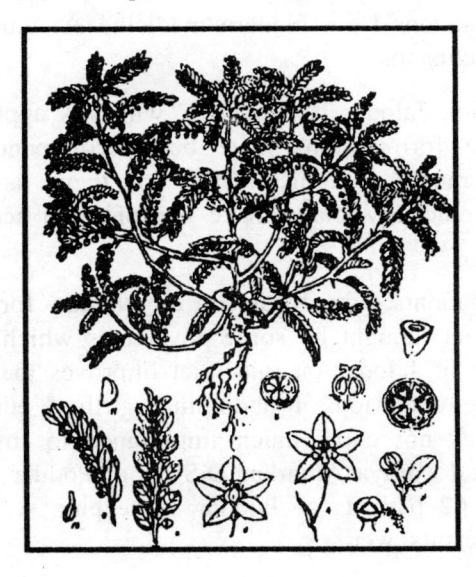

Sanskrit Name : Bhumyamalaki
Latin Name : Phyllanthus niruri

Clinical Aspects Of Liver Disorders With Reference To Jalodar.

Vd. Ajit Joshi.

Jalodar (ascites) seems to be more prevalent in all the socio-economic classes due to increasing alcohol consumption in the society. There are also a few other causes, confronted during last century for the entity Jalodar.

In my clinical practice and in hospitals during my post graduation, I have treated and observed many patients of Jalodar. They were given mainly diuretics like-lasix and were also tried tapping for no. of times as the fluid recurred. This treatment was found temporarily beneficial for lowering the abdominal girth. It's a fact that many of the Jalodar patients benefit from diuresis but there is a subset of this group which does not respond satisfactorily. I found that there is a need to obtain more information about this group. It will be extremely beneficial if physicians from modern medicine & Ayurved, work together & draw some definitive conclusions.

The main treatment for the condition Jalodar is "Virechan" which is appreciated in all the Ayurvedic texts. Many more formulations have been recommended in the Ayurvedic texts providing a wide range of choice. Each of them has its own importance by its own action. Ayurvedic physicians make use of them according to their individual skill and experience.

Ayurved also advises to put such patients on milk diet on an average for about six months [Vagbhat. chi. 15-118]. A distinct thought by some physicians which appeared for discussion was keeping the patient of Jalodar on milk diet improves the condition of 'hypoproteinemia' resulting in the regression of abdominal girth & edema. They thought that Virechana treatment does not carry much importance to improve the condition. Keeping this thought in mind Vaidya Antarkar D.S. from Poddar Ayurvedic College, Mumbai carried a study on 62 patients of Jalodar as keeping such patients on milk diet for few months. The results were,

Hepatic Disorders

In total 62-Patients :-   7 - became fluid free - 11.2%

13 - had partial absorption of fluid - 20.9%

42 - had no relief - 67.4%

In comparison with these results it will be interesting to have a look on the results which were obtained during my Ph.D. thesis work during 1991 to 1995.

I have tried 75 patients of Jalodar with virechana treatment along with milk diet. The results were as-

In total 75-Patients :-   20 became fluid free with no recurrence of fluid for 1 year - 26.6%

25 had partial absorption of fluid - 33.3%

30 patients had no-relief, discontinued or expired - 40%

This makes it clear that only milk diet is not sufficient as a treatment for the cure or relief of the Jalodar. Milk diet together with Virechana improves the condition to a great extent. Of course this claim can be made considering the clinical status of the patients. No conclusion can be drawn regarding the histological improvement in the liver as the required investigations were not carried. But it can be determined as this is the area of research & workers from Ayurved have lots of potentials in it.

In my experience there are certain limiting factors in the treatment of Jalodar.

1) Age- above 55 years

2) Liver cirrhosis

3) Abdominal Koch's & ascites due to secondaries in the liver.

Once it is cleared that milk diet & virechana together play an important role in the treatment of Jalodar, the next part of the discussion will be regarding type of milk consumed as a diet.

Properties of various types of milk have been mentioned in Ayurvedic classics e.g. Goat's milk, cow's milk, buffalo's milk etc. Cow's milk is the best choice and camel's milk or goat's milk is the next choice according to the Ayurvedic texts. Buffalo's milk is not well appreciated. Ayurved explains buffalo's milk as 'Guru'- heavy to digest whereas the other varieties like Goat's, Camel's & Cow's are 'Laghu'-easy to digest. If the molecule size of these varieties are considered, the terms Guru & Laghu can be explained on objective parameters

Here is the comparative chart of these three varieties.

	Buffalo	Cow	Goat
*C-8 -C-10 medium chain fatty acids (MCT)	3.4	6.2	17.1
*fat globules 1.5-3 micron	24.5	43.3	63.1

So cow's milk & goats milk contain C-8-C-10 medium fatty acids (MCT) at significantly higher percentage than that of buffalo which provide quicker source of energy. At the same time fat globule size is very small in cow's & goat's milk as compared to the buffalo's milk. So it will be easier for human body to digest cow's milk or goat's milk. This is a humble try to explain Ayurvedic terms guru & laghu. Interested biochemists can contribute to this hypothesis. If this hypothesis is executed with all the essential efforts and proper database is prepared then I think that all the objects explained in Ayurvedic texts as guru or laghu can be standardized properly & systematically.

I would like to highlight one more point regarding the condition cirrhosis of the liver. One can make a confirmed diagnosis of cirrhosis of the liver if it is supported with biopsy. Biopsy is not carried for every suspected cirrhotic patient by almost all the professionals. Some times it is practically not advisable. No specific curative treatment nor co-operation from patient are some of the reasons behind it.

The diagnosis is generally made with the help of L.F.T.& U.S.G. But when such information appears on academic dais then it is stamped as biased. I think if the diagnosis of cirrhosis of the liver is made with the support of distinctly disturbed L.F.T & U.S.G. then it should be accepted at academic level as a primary information or study. One who wants to undergo a detail study at higher level of academy may insist for biopsy diagnosis.

And now the last point which I would like to discuss with you about the earlier diagnosis of Jalodar or ascites. I have found in my professional practice, a symptom like 'swedavrodh' -anhidrosis which is generally associated with the symptoms of Jalodar. According to my opinion about 80% of the Jalodar patients have this symptom. If greater degree of ascites is present then this symptom does not carry much importance at later stage.

But as Ayurved explains 'samprapti' of Jalodar as,

रूद्ध्वा स्वेदाम्बुवाहानि दोषाः स्त्रोतांसि संचिताः । च.चि. १३-१८

Hepatic Disorders

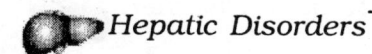

this symptom is bound to happen with the onset of Jalodar. Some times patient may appear in the clinic at the earlier stage of Jalodar. Many a times a physician may suspect evidence of Jalodar due to evidence of unhidrosis as a complication of other ailments like- Pandu ,Shoth or Grahani in due course of treatment. Even some times U.S.G study does not revel evidence of ascites but it can be suspected in the clinic. Few weeks or months later on the patient or the physician may be able to elicit the fluid thrill in the peritoneal cavity. So if the patient is having suspicious history ,with present symptoms like,

1) Loss of appetite

2) Slight increase in abdominal girth or everted Umbilicus

3) Increased debility &

4) Anhidrosis. one can suspect the condition ascites in future and can make a clinical diagnosis of Jalodar at an earlier stage.

This is possible with the knowledge of Samprapti as mentioned in Ayurvedic texts & knowledge of 'Picchavasta' which is an unique feature of Ayurved.

Dr. Ajit C. Joshi
22, Sukrawar Peth, Pune

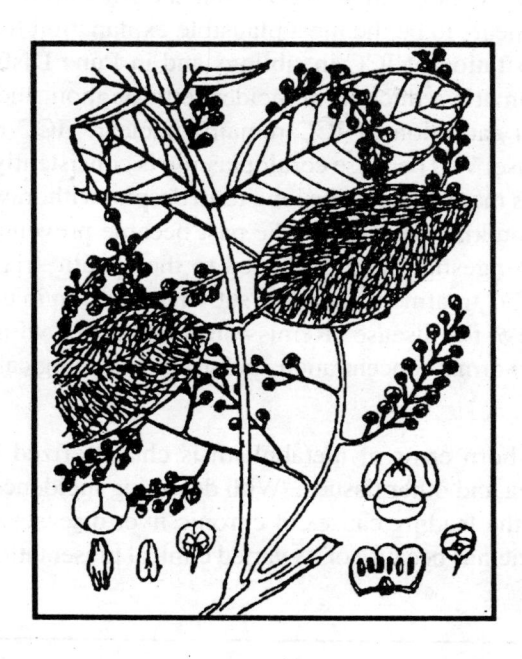

Sanskrit Name : Rohitak
Latin Name : Tecomella undulata

Hepatic Disorders

22. Copper Associated Childhood Cirrhosis

Dr. Avinash Pradhan, Dr. Shaila Bhave,
Dr. Ashish Bawadekar, Dr. Anand Pandit.

Indian Childhood Cirrhosis (ICC), Wilson's Disease (WD), Menke's Disease and Idiopathic Copper Toxicosis (ICT) are the main diseases associated with abnormal copper (Cu) Metabolism and are characterized in some by toxic accumulations of copper in the body. In Indian scenario ICC and WD has become one of the leading causes of chronic liver diseases in India.

ICC must be clearly distinguished from other chronic liver diseases including WD. ICC is associated with grossly increased hepatic, urinary and copper. These increased copper concentrations are easily demonstrated histologically with Orcein and Rhodanine staining. Environmental ingestion of copper appears to be the most plausible explanation for ICC as shown by feeding histories, the presentation of ICC in siblings and in Pune District by a change in feeding vessels and the dramatic reduction in incidence throughout India. The nature and role of a second factor in causation of ICC remains unclear. ICC dose not appear to be a straight froward early onset WD because ceruloplasmin is consistently normal and clinical and histological recovery is maintained in the long term despite withdrawal of D-penicillamine therapy. ICC, a common killer disease of the past became preventable and treatable in the early 1990s. Copper ingestion hypothesis led to therapeutic trials of the copper chelator D-Penicillamine for ICC treatment and have shown remission in upto 65% of patients in the early preicteric stage of the disease. Remission is associated with clinical recovery, reduction in hepatic copper to normal concentration, and striking histological reversal of cirrhosis.

In contrast WD an established in born error of metabolism is characterized by toxic accumulation of copper in liver, cornea and other tissues. With declining incidence of ICC Wilson's Disease has become one of the leading causes of chronic liver diseases in India. WD is peculiarly interesting for pediatricians because of its varied clinical presentation giving

Hepatic Disorders

rise to diagnostic difficulties and importantly because it is a treatable cause of liver damage and cirrhosis provided it is diagnosed early. Varied clinical presentation of WD consists of presentations like chronic liver disease, like acute or fulminant hepatitis, neuropsychiatric presentation or a symptomatic siblings. Key to diagnose WD is a high index of suspicion. Once suspected it is easy to confirm or exclude WD by appropriate tests of copper metabolism. Histology alone is not always diagnostic. Copper stains are not useful. Continuous life long drug therapy is essential in the management of WD. D-Penicillamine is still the reliable and most prescribed drug. The outcome of WD is unpredictable and changes with the clinical presentation.

Dr. Avinash Pradhan
Star Villa, Block No. 6, 917/9, Ganesh Wadi, Deccan Gymkhana, Pune – 411 004
Tel : 4457487 (O), 5651541 (R) E-mail : avipradhan@vsnl.com

Effect Of 'Stimuliv' In Viral Hepatitis

Dr. Mahesh Kagali.

Introduction

VIRAL HEPATITIS is an endemic disease in India with epidemic outbreaks, there is no specific drug for viral hepatitis. hence various modes of treatment are used in treating viral hepatitis. since long herbal medicines are used, stimmulive is one such herbal preparation, containing –

1. Kalmegh – it increases bile and gastric huice sectretion.
2. Bhringraj – reduces hepatomegaly and jaundice.
3. Pittapapda – it is a cholagogue and a mild laxative.

The syrup containing these herbal medicines Kalmegh 62.5 mg, Bhringras 200 mg, and Pittapapada 100 mg in 5 ml, was used in treating viral hepatitis and its effect on the clinical features, and laboratory parameters were studies.

Material and method

50 patients of viral hepatitis were selected with the following criteria;

- Ø Australia Antigen Negative
- Ø Not In Precoma Or Coma
- Ø Jaundice Of Less Than 6 Weeks Duration
- Ø Normal Prothrombin Time
- Ø Alkaline Phosphataese Less Than 30

25 patients were in control and 25 were in study group receiving stimuliv, 10 ml twice daily.

Hepatic Disorders

Both the groups were comparable in age, sex, biochemical abnormalities and clinical features. The patients were closely followed regards symptoms, signs, drug acceptance, drug side effects, and laboratory parameters.

The observations made were recorded in the following tables :

Table No. 1

Age and Sex Distribution in the Control group and the Stimulive group

Age in Years	Stimuliv Group		Control Group	
	Male	Female	Male	Female
11-20	2	1	0	2
21-30	9	4	8	5
31-40	3	1	5	0
41-50	2	1	1	1
50-	1	1	2	1
TOTAL	17	8	16	9

Table No. 2

Incidence of various symptoms in the Control group and the Stimuliv group

Sr. No.	Symptom	Stimuliv Group	Control Group
1.	Loss of appetite	25	25
2.	Jaundice	24	25
3.	Abdominal pain	18	23
4.	Weakness	17	15
5.	Fever	18	18
6.	Diahhrea	4	4
7.	Loss of weight	3	2
8.	Constipation	1	2
9.	Itching	2	0

Table No. 3
Mean biochemical findings in the stimuliv group and the control group on admission

Sr.no.	Biochemical Investigations	Stimulive group mean /- S.D.	Control Group Mean / - S.D.
1.	S. bilirubin	8.248 ± 4.07	8.2344 ± 3.7574
2.	S.G.O.T.	312.92 ± 108.64	332.32 ± 99.61
3.	S.G.P.T.	372.24 ± 56.44	386.60 ± 56.47
4.	S.proteins	7.3884 ± 0.9659	7.03 ± 0.762

Table No. 4
No. of patients having clay colored stools at 0, 1 and 2 weeks duration with statistical significance (X^2 test)

Duration	Stimuliv Group	Control Group	Statistical Significance
On admission	10	14	-
1 week	4	9	No
2 weeks	1	4	No

Table No. 5
No. of patients with normal biochemical findings at 4 and 5 weeks duration in both groups with statistical significance (X^2 test)

Duration	Biochemical Investigations	Stimuliv	Control	Statistical Significance
4 weeks	S. bilirubin	7	1	Yes
	S.G.O.T.	10	2	Yes
	S.G.P.T.	6	1	Yes
6 weeks	S. bilirubin	23	13	Yes
	S.G.O.T	23.	12	No
	S.G.P.T.	20	9	Yes

Hepatic Disorders

Table No. 6
No. of patients showing improvement in signs and symptoms at the end of 2 and 4 weeks with statistical significance (X^2 test)

Duration	Biochemical Investigations	Stimuliv	Control	Statistical Significance
2 weeks	Appetite	18	11	Yes
	Abd. Pain	12	4	Yes
	Jaundice	2	3	No
	Hepatomegaly	13	10	No
	Weight gain	17	9	Yes
4 weeks	Appetite	25	25	No
	Abd. Pain	16	21	No
	Jaundice	19	10	Yes
	Hepatomegaly	22	16	Yes
	Weight gain	21	17	No

Conclusion

Bed rest and good nutrition is still, the mainstay in the management of viral hepatitis, Today. However herbal drugs like kalmegh, bhringhas, and pittapapada can reduce liver cell injury or destruction, help in liver regeneration, and stimulate protein synthesis.

Dr. Mahesh Kagali
368, Nana Peth, Kagali Hospital, Pune – 411 002

Liver In Aquired Immune Deficiency Syndrome [AIDS] An Autospy Study

Dr. Sanjay D. Deshmukh, Dr. Bageshri Gogate,
Dr. S. R. Rane, Dr. S. C. Puranik, Dr. M. V. Jadhav,
Dr. Manali Ghaisas.

Key Words

Liver, Aids, HIV

Abstract

HIV is a lymphotropic virus. In the course of an infection multiple organs and organ systems are involved. Although liver is not the primary target organ of this dreaded diseases, it may show involvement by opportunistic infections, neoplasm and other AIDs related disorders. This study highlights the spectrum of hepatic abnormalities in AIDs, as encountered in autopsies. The series includes 30 complete autopsy cases of AIDs patients with detail histomorphological study of liver.

Out of these 30 cases, histological sections demonstrated lesions in 19 cases [63%], which includes, tuberculosis in 11 cases [16%], malaria in 1 case [5%], infiltration by lymphoma in 1 case [5%], disseminated erythroleukemia in 1 case [5%].

Liver was often involved as a part of disseminated primary multi systemic disorder except in the case of viral hepatitis. There were no findings specific or pathognomonic of AIDs identified in liver.

Our study highlights the association of tuberculosis and malaria in AIDs in addition to other conditions which is in contrast to reported western studies.

List of Abbreviations used in the article :

AIDS : Acquired Immunodeficiency Syndrome

TB : Tuberculosis

Hepatic Disorders

CAH : Chronic Active Hepatitis

H & E : Hematoxylin and Eosin

GMS : Gormories methanamine silver

ZN : Ziel Nielson

**Dr. Sanjay D. Deshmukh, Dr. Bageshri Gogate, Dr. S. R. Rane,
Dr. S. C. Puranik, Dr. M. V. Jadhav, Dr. Manali Ghaisas.**
Department of Pathology, B. J. Medical College & Sassoon General Hospitals, Pune, Maharashtra.

Treatment for Liver Disorders from Eye of Naturopathy

Dr.Sindhu Shiralkar

Naturopathy is not exactly a treatment – it is a way of living a healthier life. Diseases can be cured much faster by following the ways of Naturopathy. Naturopathy is a way of living which increases the energy levels of a person.

Laws of Naturopathy

The first law of Naturopathy says the reason for all dieases is the same – an unbalanced diet and an improper lifestyle.

Ayurved says that - " Yatra Sngaha kha vaigunya vyaadhi tatro pajyate"

An unbalanced diet and an improper lifestyle increases the level of toxins in our body. And an increased level of toxins gives rise to various diseases. Germs are not responsible for most of the diseases in the human body. Scientist Louis Pasteur used to believe that germs are responsible for all diseases of the human body. So, he sterilised everything before consuming it. Inspite of that, at a very young age, he suffered from high blood pressure and paralysis.

The second law of Naturopathy says that it is not the medicines which cure our diseases – it is our body which is responsible for curing the diseases. Our body energy acts on the diseases and thus the disease is cured. If the body energy levels of a person are very low, inspite of all types of medicines, he can not be cured. Our body energy is fit for fighting against germs. A balanced diet (which includes a vegetarian diet, boilded food, non-spicy food, fruits and milk) and a good life style (sufficient sleep, rest and exercises) are essential for increasing the energy levels in lur body.

Taking in to consinderation Naturopathy, we are thinking of a line of treatment for liver diseases.

Hepatic Disorders

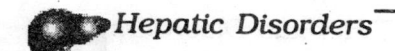

Liver is a very important organ in our body. The main fuction of liver is the secretion of bile. Bile is secreted continuously but the flow increases after eating and decreases after 8 hours. Bile secretion can be increased by practicing breathing exercises.

Digested food from the small intestines is metabolised in the liver and turned in to glycogen. Metabolism of protein, carbohydrates and fats is also done by the liver.

When a person suffers from liver diseases, metabolism is impaired. There are many kinds of liver diseases lets take Jaundice for instance. There are two types of jaundice – Infective jaundice and obstructive jaundice. Naturopathy can cure most of the liver diseases except the ones which rquire surgery.

While giving Naturopathic therapy, we take in to consideration the age of the person, general condition and digestive power of the patient. We can also take help of laboratory tests like blood test, liver function test, urine test, x-ray, sonography etc. like Ayurved, Naturppathy also believes that our bodies are made up of five elements – Earth, Water, Air, Sky & Fire. These elements are used for therapy in Naturopathy.

Importance of Earth

According to the Vedas, earth is our mother and father . 1) Earth is a very good disinfectant. 2) It creates heat and protects from cold. 3) It absorbs germs. 4) Earth contains all valuable metals in it.

In liver diseases, mud is applied on the liver area, thickmess of the application should be half an inch. The mud should be brought from the form and soaked in water the previous day.

Importance of water : Hot and cold water packs on the liver area. Seat bath is given. Water increases the blood flow to the diseased area and it improves the function of the diseased area.

Fire (heat) : A sun bath early in the morning for about half an hour is very beneficial. Drinking orange colour water is also recommended.

How to prepare

Take a glass bottle and wrap it with orange gelatin sheet. Fill it with water and keep it in the sun for 4-6 hours.

Air : Air is said to be ten times mote important than medicines. Morning walk for an hour every day supplies our bodies with oxygen and ozone. Since air is free from pollution in the mornings, it is best to take walk in mornings.

Yoga : In liver diseases, Halasana and Matsuasana, breathing exercises and meditation is a must. It increases will power and energy levels. Due to these asanas blood flow to the

Hepatic Disorders

liver is increased and the working capacity is increased.

Massage : Massage on the liver area gives stimulation to the liver cells and creates heat, improves liver function and thus get rid of the disease.

Diet therapy : Diet therapy is a very important therapy in Naturopathy. Along with the above therapy, diet therapy gives very good results.

Fast : Ayurved says "Laghanam laghu bhojanamva". In liver diseases, liver functioning is impaired. So, the liver should not be overworked. It should get some rest. At the same time, it should get nourishment. For this purpose, light diets and juices are given –

Line of treatment for a liver disease

According to the general conditions of a person, Naturopaths give instructions to the patients.

1. Morning – Lemon water which should be lukewarm or cold according to the season. Lemon is very essential for our body. It contains all types of vitamins necessary for our body. Lemon has large quantities of calcium and Vitamin C. Vitamin C cleans our body toxins. So, Naturopaths use lemon in their therapy. Start with half a lemon and increase it to 1-4 lemons in a day.

2. Enema – if bowels are not open during fasting then give lukewarm enema to the patient. Enema removes the poisons from the body.

3. Sun bath in the morning – morning walks, yogasanas, breathing exercises and meditation are absolutely essential while treating the patient. Meditation is needed because the mind of a person needs to be treated as much as the body.

4. Diet : In the beginning, we give them juices – carrot, beet and spinach. Carrot contains per 100g, 80 gm of calcium, 530mg Phosphorous, and 3150 mg of Vitamin A. Beet – in 100g, Calcium – 194 mg, Potassium – 300 mg and Phosphorous – 60 mg, Vitamin B1 – 91 mg, Oxalic Acid – 40 mg., Spinach – in 100 g, Calcium – 73 mg., Vitamin A – 9300 mg, Vitamin C – 28 mg.

A combination of these there is easy to digest and gives full food values necessary for the liver.

Another combination which is very beneficial is carrot, spinach and coconut water. Coconut water contains – 240 mg Phosporous.

In liver diseases, a patient is given lemon water 3-4 times a day and the above mentioned juices one glass at a time, according to the appetite of the patient. This is done for 3 days. After that, pure fasting in which only water is given (for 3 days). This cycle is repeated

Hepatic Disorders

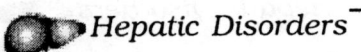

many times if necessary. Then again juices are given and then gradually diet is increased according to the appetite of the patient. Boiled vegetables, moong dal khichadi, buttermilk, cucumber, tomato, beet salad and fruits.

If accompanied by external therapy the diet therapy is very effective. Spiritual power in increased by yoga, breathing exercises and meditation and the patient is soon rid of the diseases.

Accupressure, accupuncture and magnet therapy are also included in Naturopathy.

Accupuncture is also based on the concept that our bodies are made up of five elements. And that there are 14 channels in our bodies. In Latin 'Accu' means needles and 'Pucnture' means pricking. So, Accupuncture is actually an art of healing, of curing diseases by pricking needles. There are 14 channels in our body and there is continuous energy flow in these channels. Energy is named as 'Chi' in chinese. Energy has positive and negative constituents known as ' Yin' and 'Yang' respectively. In a normal healthy person tese are balanced. When imbalance between the negative and the positive occurs, a person becomes unhealthy. In accupuncture, the obstruction in energy flows ins corrected by pricking the skin with tiny needles. There are 900 points in our bodies, out of which 8-9 points are selected for treatment.

Some Accupuncture points in liver diseases

Live 6 –7 cum superior to the tip of the medical malleolus on the medical border of tibia.

Liv 13 – on the lateral side of the abdomen below the free end of the 11th **floating rib.**

Sp 6 – 3 cum above the tip of the medical malleoulus and posterior to the border of tibia

Sp 9 – At the level of the lower border of the tibial turberosity in the depression below the lower border of the medical condyle.

Accupressure : Accupressure means the art of treating diseases by applying prssure on specific points with the help of one's thumb or with blunt ended / unpointed things. Our body has various pressure points on the palm of the hand and the soles of our feet. It is absolutely harmless and very effecting in treating chronic joint diseases.

The accupressure point for the liver is one inch below the base of the little finger on the hand and one inch below the base of the little toe on the sole of the foot.

Magnet Therapy : Magnet Therapy is becoming very popular now a days. Earth has a magnetic field and so does our body. It the magnetic field in our body. If the magnetic field in our bodyt is balanced, a person remains healthy. If there is imbalance in this magnetic field, one becomes sick. High blood pressure is controlled by using magnets. Red cells are increased in blood, cholestrol level is decreased by magnet therapy.

Hepatic Disorders

There are two types of treatments in magnet threapy - one polar and bipolar.

Every magnet has two poles - south pole and North pole.

South pole - In infections, it reduces oedema and it reduces capillary flow of blood. Vegetables and fruits remain fresh is the southern magnetic field.

North pole - It stimulates body activity. This pole has effects opposite to the south pole. Fruits ripen fast and vegetables and milk go bad in this magnetic field. While giving magnetic therapy, there should not be any wound on that part of the body. Magnetic water is also given as a part of the treating. To prepare magnetised water, fill a bottle with water and place it on a magnet for 4 - 6 hours.

Dr. Sindhu Shiralkar
Z-5, Himali Hsg. Soc., Opp. Mehendale Gaurage, Erandwane, Pune
Tel : 5461618

Hepatic Disorders

Hepatitis Induced Ascites : A Clinical Study

Vd. Ashok G. Wali,
Vd. Miss Manisha Mulye,

Introduction

Liver diseases, acute or chronic are a cause of significant human mortality. Liver diseases may results a wide variety of infections and also from various toxins. The most common infection is viral infection and amongst the toxins alcohol is the main cause of hepatitis which is found in my practice, since last 20 years. Liver disorders lead to chronic sequel such as chronic hepatitis, cirrhosis, ascites, and carcinoma.

The accumulation of fluid in the peritoneal cavity has been frequently maintained and it explained that the condition is of the nature of oedema of the cavity. The liver cirrhosis is the main etiological factor.

The successful treatment of ascites depends upon the treatment of underlying causes. Sodium restricted diet and diuretics provide symptomatic relief. However to remove the excess of fluid from the cavity, paracentesis of the abdomen is referred.1

This is no specific medicine in allopathy to treat liver disorders. Vitamin supplements and steroids are generally used to treat liver disorders in modern medicine which shows that there is no specific medicine in this developing science. The inability of modern approach to provide satisfactory answer has led physicians to search effective medicines from the herbal source. 2

Material and methods

10 patients from both sexes between age of 30-70 yrs. From all socioeconomic strata were taken for studies who were already diagnosed as Ascites according to modern science. According to Ayurveda these patients were diagnosed as "Jalodar".

In Ayurveda impaired digestive power (agni) has been considered the basic etiological

Hepatic Disorders

factor of all types of abdominal enlargements, which are producted as a result of the accumulation of excretory products. Eg. Faeces, urine, uitiated humours.

The clinical features in general include abdominal distension, weakness, sluggish, passage of faeces and flatus etc.

The eight types along with their pathogenesis and specific clinical features are given and prognosis is also mentioned. (3)

'Phalatrikadi kadha' which is used as a material for this disease. The contains and its properties are as below. (4)

Dravya	Ras	Mahabuta	Guna (General)	Guna (Specific)
Triphala	Panchras	All	Deepan Ruchya	Sar, Mehkushta har.
Guduchi	Katu	Agni vayu	Sangrahi	Swadupaki
	Tikta	Akash vayu	Ushna, Laghu	Rasayan
	Kashay	Prithwi vayu	Deepana	Daha nashak
Kutaki	Katu	Agni vayu	Ruksha laghu	Him, Bhedini
	Tikta	Akash vayu	Deepani Dahanashak	Hridya
Nimbal	Tikta	Akash vayu	Sheet laghu	Agni vatnut
	kashay	Prithwi vayu	Grahi	Ahridya
Chirait	Tikta	Akash vayu	Ruksha, Sheet Laghu	Surak Dahnut
Vasa	Tikta	Akash vayu	Laghu sheet	Vat krit
	kashay	Prithwi vayu	Kapha pitta Nashak	Hridya, kaph Pitta nashak

The kadha primarily acts on liver. Normaly liver secrets pitta which mixes with the Annaras which holps to formation of Rasa Rakta etc. dhatus.

Due to vaiety of causes the equilibrium of tridoshas is vitiated alongwith malas. Srotorodh i. e. blockage in srotas is created. Abnormal toxic dravagas which are parthiwa gather around liver to create the blockage. Secreation of Pitta is hampered. Liver is then enlarged.

Tenderness is noticed.

Triphala, Kutaki, Chirait are from Haritkyad, varga. This has qualities to clear off the abnormal doshas. Kutaki is behdini i. e. it helps to drive out the mala sanchay i. e. blocked

Hepatic Disorders

faeces is excreted. Nimbasal and vasa are from guduchyadi varga which has property to give sthirato. Guduhi and Triphala both are rasayani i. e. rejuvenative.

In short this medicine is vat – Akash Pradhan medicine. This has potential to do away with all abnormal, toxic material, blockage the liver i. e. it does shodhan karma.

As per the panchabhoutika principle ghanata is dissolved in water. In ascites, these Phalatrikadi kadha clears the obstruction and Pittamarga is cleared. Bhedan guna of kutaki prominently helpful. Triphala helps to excrete malas other ingridiets acts as pitta shoman and rasayan. 5

Dose – 20 ml BD

Timing – 6 a. m. kadha and 6. P. m. nikadha

Kadha should be prepared according to "Grantyas" diet – only milk, for some days & then other diet depending upon the results of disease.

Crietria for cure

Jalodhar is mentioned as 'Asadhya' in Ayurveda. But following crietria should be considered

1) Abdominal girth
2) Body weight
3) U. S. G. and Pathological investigations.
4) Clinical symptoms.

The final crietria for cure is as follows.

1) Report of U. S. G. shows no ascites – 100% i. e. complete relief.
2) Report of U. S. G. shows ascites – 50% i. e partial relief.
3) Report of U. S. G. shows huge ascites – i. e. 0% no relief.

Observations

Classification according to 'Sex'

Male	Female	Total
7	3	10
(70%)	(30%)	(100%)

Hepatic Disorders

Classification according to 'Age'

Age gr.	Male	Female	Total
40-50	2 (20%)	1 (10%)	3 (30%)
51-60	4 (40%)	2 (20%)	6 (60%)
61-70	1 (10%)	0 (0%)	1 (10%)
Total	7 (70%)	3 (30)	10 (100%)

Details of history, clinical examination and other revelant observations of patients were recorded in the proforma specially sesigned for the research.

Classification according to 'abd girth'

Length in cm	Male	Female	Total
81-90	3	2	5
91-100	1	0	1
100 – 110	0	1	1
111 – 120	2	0	2
121 – 130	1	0	1
Total	7 (70%)	3 (30%)	10 (100%)

Classification according to 'Weight'

Wt. in kgs	Male	Female	Total
41-50	1	1	2
51-60	0	1	1
61-70	0	1	1
71-80	4	0	4
81-90	1	0	1
91-100	1	0	1
Total	7 (70%)	3 (30%)	10 (100%)

Classification according to 'History' :

	Alcohol	Non-Alcohol	Veg.	Non-veg
Male	6	1	16	6
Female	1	2	0	3
Total	7 (70%)	3 (30%)	1 (10%)	9 (90%)

Hepatic Disorders

Discussion :

There are 70% male patients while 30% are female patients suffered from ascites. It is seen that male patients are more proune to this diesease.

There are 6 patients out of 10 are in the category of 51-60 age and again male are more dominant in this age group. I. e. 40%. It is followed by 3 patients in the category of 41-50 age. Again male are dominant i. e. 20%. In general 41-60 is the prone age group for this disease.

If we observed the abdominal girth it seems that 50% of patients are in the group of 81-90 c. m. and is followed by 20% in the category of 111 – 120 c. m. The highest abdominal girth is seen in one patient i. e. 121 – 130 c. m.

According to body wieght 40% patients are in the category of 71 – 80 kg. and is followed by 20% patients in 421 – 50 kg. There is one patient in the highest category of the wt. i. e. 91 – 1000 kg.

If we look the history of patients all patients have a history of 'Jaundice' (Hepatitis) Non – vegeterian and alcoholic patients are more prone to this diesease i. e. 90 % and 70% respectively.

Results :

The patients showing following signs & symptoms are said to be improving.

1) Reducing the abdominal girth.
2) Reducing the body weight.
3) Liver function tests should be normal.
4) Clinically oedema is totally absent.
5) Quantity of stool and urine should be increased.
6) Liver & spleen should be palpable.
7) Comparision of before & after treatment U. S. G. Reports.

Classification of patients according to Relief :

	Male	Female	Total
Complete Relief	2	0	2
Partial Relief	2	0	2
No Relief (Patient expired)	3	3	6
Total	7(70%)	3(30%)	10(100%)

Conclusion :

In the present study it was observed that the Ayurvedic medicine 'Phaltrikadi Kadha' of Sharangadhar may reduce the severity of disease and may help in prevention of complications in such cases. There is 20% total cure who are young and the disease is in the first step so with the help of pathyapthya and phaltrikadi kadha. Patients are totally cured. 20% patients having partial relief and they are tin under treatment. The results in these patients are hopeful, because they are symptomless. 60% patients are not cured. Out of this 6 patients 3 patients are very much serious before starting the treatment. Ingeneral these 6 patients are expired within 6-7 months of treatment, because of seriousness of the illness, irregular pathyapathya and medicine.

It is noticed that the alcoholic liver cirrohosis which is the main cause of ascites and is not curable. At the same time non - veg eterian are also not curable. Without history of alcohol and the vegeterians are likely to be curable. The pathyapathya plays the most important role in this disease.

References :

1) Davidson stendey and Macleod John : The Principles and practice of Medicine (Longman group ltd. 1971 5th E. L. B. S. edition, published 1973).

2) Jamkhedkar, Sigh, Ashelesha : Clinical trial of Activ fort in Acute Hepatitis Journal of NIMA, Jully 1998, P. G.

3) Singhal G. D., Tripathi S. N., Sharma K. R. : Ayurvedic Clinical Dignosis based on Madhava – Nidan (Delhi : Chaukhmba Sanskrut Pratishtan, 1985).

4) Datar A. W. : Vanaspaticne swabhav Arthat Gunadharma Shastra (Bombay : A. V. Datar, 1966).

5) Haldavanekar S. K. : Twenty medicines of panchbhoutik chikista (Sangli : P. C. S. K. 1999).

Vd. Ashok G. Wali,
Vd. Miss Manisha Mulye,
'Prakruti', Panchabhoutik chikistalaya, Rajrampuri, 3rd Lane, Kolhapur (M. S.), India.

Role of Yakrit : Ayurvediya Vivechana.

Vd. Darsha Tilay

The origin & development of the word Yakrit is य म् अ कृ : य संयम करोति

The meaning is that the liver controls various physiological events.

Liver can have various diseases as described in Ayurved i.e. Yakritdalyodar, Yakritvidradhi etc.

In these diseases there is a specific treatment for liver. But there are many other diseases in which there is no direct relation of liver, still we have to consider it in our treatment.

In this paper, I am trying to explain this importance of liver in various diseases other than liver itself. Here 'why & how is this consideration important?' will be discussed.

In Brihattrayi, following references regarding liver are directly available.

ORIGIN OF LIVER

गर्भस्य यकृत्प्लीहानौ शोणितजौ । सु.शा. ४/२७

POSITION OF LIVER

हृदयस्य अधो दक्षिणत: यकृत् सु.शा. ४/३१२

SITE OF BLOOD

शोणितस्य स्थानं यकृत्प्लीहानौ । सु.शा. २९/१६

RAKTAVAHA SROTAS

रक्तवहे द्वे तयोर्मूलं यकृत्प्लीहानौ रक्तवाहिन्यश्च धमन्य: । सु.शा. ९/१८

LIVER: AN ABDOMINAL ORGAN

Hepatic Disorders

पंचदश कोष्ठांगानि तद्यथा — यकृच्च । सु.शा. ९/१२

SITE OF RANJAK PITTA

यत्तु यकृत्प्लीहनो: पित्त तस्मिन् रंजकोऽग्निरिति संज्ञा । सु.सू. २९/१०

RAKTADHARA KALA

द्वितीया रक्तधरा नाम मांसस्य अभ्यन्तरत:

तस्यां शोणितं विशेषतश्च सिरासु

यकृत्प्लीहनोश्च भवन्ति । सु.शा. ९/१२

PURISHADHARA KALA

यकृत्समन्तात: कोष्ठं च तथान्त्राणि समाश्रिता ।

उण्डुकस्थ विभजते मलं मलधरा कला ॥ सु.शा. ४/१७

Yakritdalludar   च.चि. १३/३२

Abhyantar yakrit vidradhi   च.सू. १७/८२

Raktapitta   च.चि. ४/१०

In Charakadi granthas there is clear relation of yakrit in these diseases.

Hence giving the explanation on the importance of yakrit in the same will be repetition & subject expanding.

The role of yakrit is explained as relation of yakrit with dosha, dhatu & mala.

Dosha & yakrit

Ranjak pitta is situated in liver. In any liver disorder due to adhar-adheya sambandha the function of rasa ranjana will be disturbed. Also if there is vitiation of ranjak pitta, it will affect liver. In normal condition,

स खलु आप्यो रस: यकृत्प्लीहनो प्राप्यरामुपैति । सु.सू. १४/४

रञ्जितास्तेजसात्वाप: शरीरस्थेन देहिनाम् ।

अव्यापन्ना प्रसन्नेन रक्तमित्यभिधीयते ॥ सु.सू. १४/७

Hepatic Disorders

Ranjak pitta: Contribution In Digestion

Acharya Vagbhata had described the site of ranjaka pitta as amapakvashaya. Pitta from liver enters in gastrointestinal tract through a channel. Though this hepatobiliary system is well explained in modern medicine there are few references in Ayurved regarding it.

कालखण्डग्न नलिकामध्यगतजलं पित्तम् । सु.क. ९/४७ डल्हण

पित्तं कालखण्डगम् । सु.सू. २९/९३ डल्हण

In bahupitta & ruddhapatha kamala, if one studies the symptoms thoroughly there is alpagni (less digestion) in ruddhapatha type. When the obstruction reduces hunger starts increasing. Thus ranjak pitta in liver helps in digestion. In the other way one had to take in account this role of liver in agnimandyaja vikar.

Dhatu & Yakrit

Blood vessels from liver supply whole body. Through this route only, the function jeevankarma takes place.

तेषां रसादिधातूनां क्षयवृद्धि शोणितनिमित्ते । सु.सू. १४/२१

There is a reference that blood is responsible for vriddhi & kshaya of other rasadi dhatus. Hence, it is necessary that the role of liver, the moolasthana of raktavaha srotas should be considered in increase & decrease of other dhatus.

Rasa & Yakrit

When there is vitiated rasadhatu, poshya raktadhatu will also get vitiated & then rasa to rakta conversion place, yakrit will also get affected.

Pandu is a disease of rasavaha srotas. In pandu, where there are many reasons that increase pittadosha, it causes burning (vidaha) in rakta & mansa. Therefore there is damage of liver tissue.

कुक्षे: दक्षिणभागरथानरथ मांसखण्डम् तत्पर्याय कालखंजम् - यकृत् । अमरकोष

Rakta & Yakrit

Almost in all diseases of blood, one has to treat liver, because liver & spleen are the only organs that control the other sthanas of blood.

तत्रस्थमेव यकृत्प्लीहानौ शेषणां

शोणितस्थानानामनुग्रहं करोति । सु.सू. २९/९६

Mamsa –Medadi & Yakrit

रसाद्रक्तं ततो मांसं मांसान्मेदस्ततोऽस्थिच ।

अस्थ्नो मज्जा तत: शुकं शुकात् गर्भ: प्रसादजा : ।। च.चि. १४/९६

By this, the first dhatu formed from ahararasa is rasa. From that rakta is derived, from rakta, mamsa & the process continues. If there is samata (undigested contents) in the first rasa dhatu, the next raktamamsadi dhatus will also become sama which will cause apatarpanajanya diseases. Here acts ranjakagni, if liver is normal functioning this ama gets digested & further pathology is prevented. After this digestion in liver, there is only action of dhatwagni & no support of pachak & ranjakagni.

यत्तु यकृत्प्लीहनो पित्तं तारिमन रंजकोग्निः इति संज्ञा । सु.सू. २९/९०

Though there is a reference—

अग्निरेव शरीरे पित्तान्तर्गतः कुपिताकुपितः शुभाशुभानि करोति । च.सू. १२/११

Only pachaka & ranjaka pitta are called agni in charakadi texts directly. Thus here we see the special digestion due to this not only raktavikriti but also mamsa medadi dhatu vikriti are prohibited.

Mala & Yakrit

Pitta from liver comes in pakwashaya & gives color to stool. If there is obstruction in this way, like in ruddhapatha kamala, stool becomes clay coloured. Here one can understand the field of purishadhara kala in liver. When the obstruction is removed the fecal matter becomes normal in color due to pitta.

स्वस्थानमागते पित्ते पुरीषे पित्तरंजिते । च.चि. १६/१३१

By Ayurvedic concept, urine is formed in pakwashaya. The ranjak pitta as said above, comes in pakwashaya & gives a faint yellowish tinge to urine. In diseases like uddhapatha kamala the pitta due to obstruction is expelled from its site & circulates all over the body. As function of urine is kledavahana, the urine becomes high colored due to increase in pitta circulation.

Pranavaha Srotas & Yakrit

In the causative factors of pranavaha srotas, as explained in charaka viman 5, there is स्रोतांस्यन्यैश्च दारुणे i.e. violations of other srotasas. In yakritvidradhi, there is a symptom dyspnoea. It can be explained like this In the process of respiration, the pranavayu get spread in all over the body through blood & thus does the jeevaniya function.

प्राणो हि शोणितं अनुवर्त्तते

When there is pathology in blood, it affects the inspiration & expiration process, hence the symptom dyspnoea develops.

Also the development of liver & lungs, blood is the basic constituent. This reference also supports the above explanation.

Hepatic Disorders

Annavaha Srotas & Yakrit

As described in ranjak pitta & yakrit, liver helps in digestion.

Udakavaha Srotas & Yakrit

It is not directly related with liver but kloma, which is just below the liver very closely, situated, is pipasasthana & so related to liver.

क्लोम कालखंडादधस्तात् स्थितं दक्षिणपार्श्वस्थं तिलकं प्रसिद्धम् । सु.नि. ९/१८ डल्हण

क्लोम्नि पिपासा । सु.नि. ९/२२

Miscelleneous
Amapakwashaya & yakrit

In the description of urdhwaga & adhoga raktapitta, it is said

आमाशयात्त्वजदूर्ध्वमधः पक्वाशयाद्व्रजेत् ।

विदग्धयोर्द्वयोश्चापि द्विधाभागं प्रवर्तते ।

केचित् सयकृतः प्लीहनः प्रवदन्त्यसृजो गतिम् ॥ सु.सू. ४५/५-६

यद्यपि रक्तस्य यकृत्प्लीहस्थानत्वात् आमपक्वाशयाभ्यां प्रवर्तन न सम्भवति तथापि

प्रकुपितं रक्तस्य तत्रापि गमनात् प्रवर्तनं ताभ्यामेव सम्भवत्येव । डल्हण

This means liver & spleen being site of blood, supplies gastrointestinal trac. In normal condition there is no bleeding through these sites. Here we can understand the role of bastichikitsa in liver diseases. As blood is in liquid form & circulates all over the body, it also explains the action of bastichikitsa in almost all diseases in the body.

Toxins & yakrit

Garavisha, a special type of toxin described in Ayurved, affect liver & hepatomegaly may take place.

नानाप्राण्यंगशमलविरुद्धौषधिमरस्मनाम् ।

विषाणां चाल्पवीर्याणां रोगो गर इति स्मृतः ।

तेन पाण्डु कृशोल्पग्निः

महोदरयकृत्प्लीह । अ/ह. उत्तर ३५/४०-४२

The reason for hepatomegaly is that blood had special affinity towards toxins. The toxins immediately get spread in the body through blood.

Hepatic Disorders

Hridroga & yakrit

According to Acharya Bhargava, as mentioned in Kashyapasamhita in development of different organs in fetus, from blood, heart & liver are developed.

शोणितात् हृदयं तस्य जायते हृदयात् यकृत् ।

यकृतो जायते प्लीहा प्लीहन: फुफुसमुच्यते ।

परस्परनिबध्दानि सर्वाण्येतानि भार्गव ॥   का.सं. शारीर - गर्भविक्रान्ति

In many patients hepatomegaly as a result of certain heart disease like LVF are seen in practice. With other explanations the above reference supports the pathology.

Dr. Darsha S. Tilay (M. D. Scholar)
437, Budhwar Peth, Pune – 411 002, Tel : 4455976 (R)

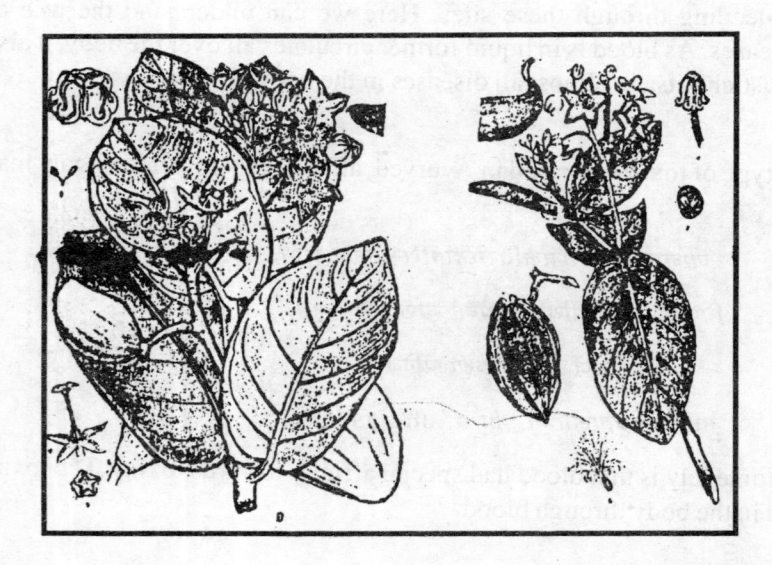

Sanskrit Name : Arka
Latin Name : Calotrpis procera

Hepatic Disorders

28. Yakrddalyudara - Samprapti & Chikitsa

Dr. Monica Vanarase

Due to brief describing style in Ayurveda, the total description regarding samprapti of a vyadhi is hard to get. Out of 8 varieties of udara, 'Pleehodara' is one variety. The manifestation of Yakraddalyudara is same as Plihodara.

एसमेव यकृदपि दक्षिणपार्श्वस्थं कुर्यात् ।

तुल्यहेतुलिङ्गोषधत्वात् तस्य प्लीहजठर एवावरोध इति ॥ C.Chi. 13/38.

Here, we will consider manifestation of Swatantra Yakrddalyudara.

Plihodara - Samprapti

वामपार्श्वाश्रितः प्लीहा च्युतः स्थानात् प्रवर्धते ।

शोणितं वा रसादिभ्यो विवृद्धं तं विवर्धयेत् ॥

C.Chi. 13/36.

There are 2 clauses i) च्युतः स्थानात् प्रवर्धते

ii) शोणितं वा रसादिभ्यो विवृद्धं तं विवर्धयेत् ।

i) च्युतः :- Spleen gets displaced

ii) Spleen gets enlarged due to increase in quantity of rakta or increase in the quantity of Rasadi dhatus.

These causative factors are considered for Yakrut-vrddhi.

Lets discuss Second causative factor.

Hepatic Disorders

ii) Shonitavrddhi - This can be elicitated by samprapti of Raktapitta.

तै: हेतुभि: समुत्क्लिष्टं पित्तं रक्तं प्रपद्यते ।
तद्योनित्वात् प्रपन्नं च वर्धते तत् प्रदूषयत् ।
तस्योष्मणा द्रवो धातु धातोर्धातो: प्रसिच्यते ।
स्विद्यतस्तेन संवृद्धिं भूयस्तदधिगच्छति ॥   C.Chi. 4/7,8.
प्लीहानं च यकृच्चैव तदधिष्ठाय वर्तते ।
स्रोतांसि रक्तवाहीनि तन्मूलानि हि देहिनाम् ।   C.Chi 4/10.

Causative factors
⇩
Accentuation of pitta.
⇩
Reaches to Rakta (as it takes origin from it)
⇩
pitta vitiates rakta
⇩
pitta further aggravated
⇩
Heat of pitta - Liquid fraction of rakta pervades one dhatu to other dhatu
⇩
Due to 'Oushnya' - There is an exudation of more of liquids from dhatus.
⇩
Liquid mixed with pitta
⇩
pitta & rakta - increased.
⇩
Site is Raktavaha Srotasa

Thus Yakrutvrddhi due to Shonitavraddhi

ii) Consider Second Cause -

रसादिभ्यो विवृद्धं तं विवर्धयेत् ।

The term 'रसादिभ्यो' indicates rasa, mansa, meda, asthi

Hepatic Disorders

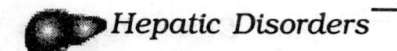

Here vitiation of Rasa is important.

Consider the general samprapti of Udara

रुध्वा स्वेदाम्बुवहानि दोषाः स्रोतांसि संचिताः ।

प्राण अग्निअपानान् संदूष्य जनयन्ति उदरं नृणाम् ॥ C.Chi. 13/20.

Accumulated dosas obstruct Swedavaha & Udakavaha Srotasas & vitiate Prana, Apana, Agni(samana) as a result of which udara is manifested.

As samana gets vitiated there is vitiation of swedavaha & ambuvaha srotasas because samana regulates these two.

स्वेददोषाम्बुवाहानि स्रोतांसि समाधिष्ठितः ।

अन्तरग्नेश्च पार्श्वस्थ समानोऽग्निबलप्रदः ॥ C.Chi. 28/8.

Also there is vitiation of prana & Apana. Hence Poorana(by prana) Vivek(by samana)Dharana(by Apana) get disturbed leading to again accumulation of dosas.

Accumulation

⇩

Srotorodha

⇩

Vimargagamana

⇩

Udara

So, 'Udara' has this specific nature of samprapti. Without vitiation of samana Udara is not possible.   Vitiation of Samana - Rasa vitiates

Rasa contributes to snehana, dharan, tarpana of the body. It gets converted into 'Rakta' in Raktavaha Srotas. This 'Rakta' will be responsible for growth of body elements.

तेषां क्षयवृद्धि शोणितनिमित्ते   Su.s. 14/21.

Hence vitiation of rasa

⇩

vitiation of rakta

⇩

vitiation of other dhatus.

Also according to Charaka,

तेषा प्रकोपात् स्थानस्थाव मार्गगाश्च शरीरधातवः

प्रकोपमापदयन्ते, इतरेषां प्रकोपाद् इतराणि च ।

Hepatic Disorders

स्रोतांसि स्रोतांसि एव धातवश्च धातूनेव प्रदूषयन्ति प्रदुष्टाः ।
तेषां सर्वेषामेव वातपित्तश्लेष्माण प्रदुष्टा दूषयितारो भवन्ति, दोषस्वभावादिति   C.Vi. 5/9

Vitiation of srotasas ro dhatus spread from one to other.

Vitiation of Dhatvagni leads to dhatupradosaj vikara.

Considering these factors -

Vitiated rasa due to 'samana' vitiation
⇩
Moves all over body.
⇩
If Dhartagni of Mansa & Rakta vitiation is there, the rasa gets stagnated in Yakrut
⇩
The elements of Mansa - Guru, Sthira, Kathin in vitiated rasa will cause Yakrutvraddhi
⇩
मांसज यकृतवृद्धि

On examination of abdomen, this Yakrut will be hard to feel.

Charaka stated plihavrddhi as कठीण , कच्छपंसरस्थान्

Thus, firstly vrddhi is hard & then like कच्छपंसरस्थान् & i.e. stony hard.

This 'Stony hardness' will be due to 'Asthijanya Yakrutvrddhi'

Dhatu	Panchabhautikatva	Properties
Rasa	Jala	Drava, Mrudu etc.
Rakta	Agneya	Drava, Mrudu, chala etc.
Mansa	Parthiv	Sthoola, Guru, Manda
Meda	Jala & Prithvi	Sthir, Kathin
Asthi	Parthiv ++	Guru Khara Kathina, Sthira

Thus the 'Vimargagaman' of the rasa, Mansa, Meda etc. can be possible & can be understood by the shape, consistency of Yakrut on abdominal examination & symptoms of the patient.

In this case treatment will be according to 'Dhatupradosaja Vikara'.

Guiding principles of Yakrutvrddhi Treatment :

i) Rasajanya - Tikta rasa, Langhan, Pachana

Hepatic Disorders

ii) Raktajanya - Same as Raktapitta

                           Virechana

                           Raktasruti

iii) Mansajanya - शस्त्रक्षाराग्निकर्म च   C.Chi. 28

iv) Medojanya - Karshana

v) Asthijanya - tikta rasa, Tikta ghrita, Basti (C.Chi. 28)

         जन्मनैवोदरं सर्वं प्रायः कृच्छतमं मतम् ।

बलिनस्तदजाताम्बु यत्न साध्यं नवोत्थितम् ॥ C.Chi. 13/54.

All varities of Udara are difficult to cure in Jatodakavashta

         Srotorodha

         Dosapak

         Jatodakavastha

In such cases, considering 'virechana' treatment, drug selection will be according to affected dhatus, bala of patient, kala(Ritu) etc.

Selection of drug according to dhatu -

Dhatu	Drug
Rasajanya	Aragvdha
Raktajanya	Trivrut
Mansajanya	Trivrut Leha
Medojanya	Kalyanaka 1
Medojanya	Satala etc.

Thus, like Plihodara, Yakruddalyudara samprapti is discussed.

This will bcontribute to specific course of ' स्वतंत्र यकृद्दाल्युदर '.

Vd. Monika R. Vanarase
C-17, Panchratneshwar Soc., Near Modak Vihir, Next to Keshav Complex, Dhanakwadi, Pune – 411 043 Tel : 4375925

Liver Disorders and Their Ayurvedic Management

Vaidya Vilas Nanal

Liver disorders are not a rarity anymore. As an Ayurvedic physician one is required to treat liver disorders much more often than naught. An elaborate description of either the organ liver and spleen or their role in physiology or pathology is not clearly described by the ancient authors. Hence one has to make use of Tantra Yukti and understand the underlying mechanism.

Before considering anything we shall consider the epistemological aspect of the organ under consideration. The word Yakrut has two verbs in it

1 Ya is derived from a root indicating activity, mobility. इण् गतौ धातो:

2 Krut is derived from either of the following two verbs कृतिदिने to break down, disintegrate or डुकृञ् करणे to be instrumental in performing any activity.

Hence that organ of the body, which is engaged in continuous activity of breaking down various stimuli, these could be food, water, air or other sensory stimuli is called Yakrut. Or that organ of the body, which is instrumental in sustaining life process.

This definition of Yakrut would explain the vital role played by the liver in the physiological as well as pathological states.

Ayurveda describes the organ YAKRUT as the *Mula Sthana* of the *Raktavaha Srotas*. This is the site where the Yakrut takes up the *Ahara rasa* and the conversion begins. This lasts for next five and one-quarter days (3015 Kalas). At the end of, which Rasa is converted to Rakta proper, Mala Pitta, Upa dhatu Sira Kandara, Sukshma Mamsa and finally Ojus. Thus converted Rakta is capable of providing the Jeevana by its Spanda attribute.

Site in the abdominal cavity it is situated in the right upper quadrant inferolaterally to the heart, under the diaphragm and covered by the ribcage.

Hepatic Disorders

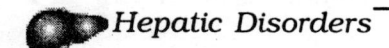

Extent - mainly on the right side of the abdominal cavity with an extension on the left.

Relations

Superior Diaphragm (Maha Prachira Peshi) covers the superior surface completely.

Superior Base of right lung (Dakshina Phupphusa) in case of Yakrut Vidradhi Shwasa is a major / cardinal sign.

Superior, medially Heart (Hrudaya) in case of Raktapitta Hrudi Atulya Peeda or an acute sharp pain in the heart region is described.

Medially Stomach (Jathara) the left lobe of liver extends to it.

Inferior Hepatic Flexure of the ascending colon (Arohi Bruhat Antra). In cases of Purishaja Udavarta pain in the hepatic regions is commonly seen which is relieved by defecation.

Inferior Gall Bladder (Pittashaya) responsible for imparting the *Tyakta Drava Awastha* to Pitta by concentration by reabsorption of it. In cases of Vidagdha Ajirna, Amla Pitta we have this dilute Drava Bahula Pitta leading to Utklesha, Chhardi, Drava Mal etc.

Inferior loops of Small Intestine (Pachyamanashaya) or Grahani.

Posterior Rt. Kidney (Vrukka) this is the third direction of Rasa Samvahana – the Shabda or Tiryak Gati.

Ayurvedic Embryological consideration according to Sushruta and Vagbhatta the Yakrut is derived from the Accha portion of the fetal blood. It means that the blood fraction, which gives rise to the liver is clear, fluid in nature. Hence the structure is soft, well organized and secretory in nature. It secretes Pachaka Pitta that is stored in the Pittashaya or the Gall bladder. The liver can and does secrete more than 500cc of Pitta. This is stored in the gall bladder and reabsorbed till only a fraction of original Pitta remains. Vagbhatta calls this as Tyakta Drava Pitta. The concentration is of vital import. If this concentration is altered it leads to a lot of diseases arising out of Agni Vaishamya. We have two sets of properties in Dosha Pitta viz. Laghu, Ushna, Tikshna, Sukshma on one hand while on the other a set of Drava, Sasneha and Sara Gandha being common to both. If the dilution in the gall bladder is more we have Drava predominant signs like nausea, vomiting, fever etc. while if the concentration is to high then Ushna and Tikshna predominant signs emerge like burning, thirst, sweat, giddiness hemorrhage etc.

Out of the causes enumerated of Pitta vitiation Madya or consumption of alcohol is by far the most common. Mádya is described as an antagonist of Ojus substantially (Dravyatah), qualitatively (Gunatah) as well as functionally (Karmatah). Ojus is responsible for holding Dhatus together (*Deha Sthiti Nibandhana*) while Madya tends to render them loose (*Sura Swabhavat Eva Jarjari Karoti*). Alcohol if consumed according to the Vidhi laid down then

Hepatic Disorders

it causes minimum damage. But if it is consumed on excess or not in conformity with the sequence then the consequences are not favorable. Madya like Ahara can be Amrut if taken timely and in moderation, keeping in mind time, constitution and habits. If consumed with disregard to these the result is disease.

Let us consider the various effects that alcohol consumption can bring about.

1 Agni Mandya alcohol is liquid and consumed in large amount without consideration to age, homologation, season; constitution etc. leads to an environment that is predominantly liquid. Cold, liquid intake leads to slowing down of Agni. The assorted snacks taken with alcohol are Pungent, Salty and Oily. This combination is potentially harmful to the liver because the ice or very cold liquid taken with spicy articles leads to enhanced production of Pitta. Increased and acute demand results in qualitative compromise resulting in indigestion of the Guru substances invariably consumed with it. Large amount of Drava leads to Rakta, Meda and Majja Dhatu vitiation while the spicy, salty and oily substances vitiate Meda and the heavy substances contaminate the Mamsa. These leads to a Sannipata characterized by Pitta and Kapha enhancement and comparatively depleted Vayu. Associated by contaminated Rasa, Rakta, Mamsa, Meda, Majja and finally Ojus.

अजनाद् अजीर्णादति जनात् विषमाशनात्
असात्म्यगुरुशीतातिरूक्षसइदुष्ट जनात्
दुष्यति अग्निः स दुष्टः अन्नं न तत् पचति लघ्वपि
अपच्यमानं शुक्तत्वम् यात्यन्नं विषरूपताम् । च.चि. १५/४४
२ तथान्नमपि तेनैव अग्निना पक्वममृततां याति अपक्वं विषरूपताम् । अ.स.शा. ६

the ingested food if digested properly is like Amruta while if not digested properly then it exhibits toxic results. Now if we have to relate this to the alcohol intake it could be as under

Avidhi Madya Pana	Excessive Alcohol intake taken too fast leads to ADH – NADH – NAD axis abnormality this leads to
Agnimandya due to large amount of liquid	Acetaldehyde production, which is highly toxic
Madya Apaka leading to Shuktata	Manifesting as liver disorder
Visha sadrush parinama	Alcohol induced hepatopathy.
Involvement of Yakrut and other Dhatus leading to grave disorders including those of Ojus.	

3 Madya and Pachaka Pitta interaction.

As seen before the Gall bladder has an important role to play in concentration of Pitta.

Hepatic Disorders

Pachaka Pitta is said to of Pancha Mahabhautika in constitution, but with a distinct shift in the favor of Agni.

Agni Ushna, **Tikshna**, Laghu Vayu Sara, Laghu Jala Sara, Drava, Sasneha Akasha Laghu, Prithvi **Visra**.

Looking at this set of qualities the Agni predominance is obvious but at the same time contribution from other Mahabhootas is also important. Due to Jala it can spread evenly and form a thin film covering the whole surface, the low unctuousness imparts penetrability and the lightness to penetrate deep in the cells and bring about conversion *Pilu Paka*. Samana Vayu is instrumental in this process of food break down, carriage of first nutrient to the heart for circulation. Since Samana is more subtle than Pitta it cause its secretion and reabsorption at appropriate time.

Amla Rasa or the Sour taste is known to generate Pitta in the body, Madya is sour in taste and post digestive effect (Vipaka). It also has affinity for the Meda or the adipose tissue and Rakta and it renders the body tissues lax hence prone to accumulation and occlusion.

सर्वेषाम् मद्यमम्लानामुपर्युपरितिष्ठति च.चि. २४/११६

अम्लं अति उपयुज्यमानम् तर्षयति, संमीलयत्यक्षिणी, कफं विम्लापयति
पित्तम् वर्धयति, रक्तं दूषयति, मांसं विदहति, कायं शिथिलीकरोति, परिदहति कंठमुरोहृदय च
च.सू. २६/४३-१

Excessive consumption of sour taste leads to thirst, difficulty in keeping eyes open, liquefies Kapha, increases and vitiates Pitta substantially, qualitatively and functionally as well. It also contaminates Rakta, Mamsa and renders the body lax and prone to other diseases along with heartburn.

Therefore excessive alcohol consumption leads to vitiation of Pitta and Samana all the way manifesting as Rakta, Mamsa, Meda, Shukra and Ojus.

4 Alcohol consumed instead of food. Vagbhatta describes correct time for food consumption as under

प्रसृष्टे विण्मूत्रे हृदि सुविमले दोषे स्वपथगे
विशुद्धे च उद्गारे क्षुदुपगमने वाते अनुसरति
तथा अग्नौ उद्रिक्ते विशदकरणे देहे च सुलभौ
प्रयुंजीत आहारं विधिनियमितं काल: स हि मत: अ/ह/सू ८/५५

This is a peculiar physiological state characterized by timely evacuation, acuity and alertness of sense organs, clear eructation, sense of hunger, unobstructed flatus, Agni stimulated and ready, lightness in the body, Vata, Pitta and Kapha in their respective sites. Kapha in the

Hepatic Disorders

Amashaya /stomach, Pitta in the Grahani / small intestine and Vayu in the Pakwashaya / large intestine. In such a condition if alcohol is consumed it affects all these factors adversely giving rise to liquefaction of Kapha, precipitates Pitta and causes irritation to the Shleshmadhara Kala leading to conditions like Amla Pitta, Parinama Shoola, Grahani. This contaminated Ahara Rasa is absorbed from the gut by Samana and taken to Hrudaya for circulation and from there on to various Srotomulas. These in turn get vitiated and depending upon the type of Madya exhibit different signs and symptoms.

5 Oka Satmya of Madya and Liver (effect of habitual and chronic alcohol intake).

When a person consumes alcohol regularly and in more than moderate amount, his body gets accustomed to a certain amount of alcohol level. Sour taste is responsible for generation and secretion of Pitta. Among all the sour articles Madya is the most potent and foremost. Alcohol when consumed causes secretion of Pitta, chronic alcoholic cannot secrete Pitta without alcohol. Hence in a situation where alcohol intake is suddenly reduced or cut off the Pitta generated in the Liver does not find a way to the gut for want of stimulus. Owing to the Ushna and Tikshna attributes of accumulated Pitta in the liver it tends to undergo physiological / functional changes like Yakrut Paka (inflammation), Yakrut Vruddhi (Hepatomegaly), Rakta Vaha Srotovibandha (obstruction to the flow of Pitta). This leads to manifestation of Kamala (jaundice) this is a result of Pitta Vimarga Gamana. If the person starts consuming alcohol again the result is much more serious due to accentuation of Pitta.

On this background we shall now consider some of the more commonly encountered alcohol induced liver disorders viz.

Yakrut Paka

Medomaya Yakrut and

Yakrut Shosha

Let us consider their Samprapti from the Ayurvedic point of view.

As we have seen before that Madya has an affinity for Pitta and Kapha. Similarly it has a peculiar affinity for Rakta, Meda and Ojus too. Hence when Madya is consumed with disregard to the prescribed method it leads to involvement of one or more of the above constituents and Agni and the respective srotas. Paka is a result of vitiated Pitta, Kapha and Rakta, Medomayata of liver is result of Meda and Kapha vitiation while Shosha is a product of increased Vayu and depleted body Dhatus. Ayurveda classifies Madya as Tikshna or strong beverages and Saumya or mild varieties.

Yakrut Paka

Those alcoholic beverages having a high concentration of Ethanol in them possess Ushna, Tikshna, Vyavayi and Vikasi attributes. In the country liquors in order to enhance the kick

Hepatic Disorders

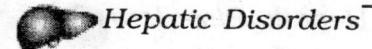

some toxic materials are used, owing to their toxicity the Vyavayi and Vikasi activity is enhanced. Strong liquors tend to vitiate Pitta all the way i.e. Dravyatah, Gunatah and Karmatah too. Vitiated Pitta brings about liquefaction of the local tissues this leads to diseases like Amla Pitta, Amashaya Shotha, Chhardi, Parinama Shoola, Grahani etc.

Drinking on the rocks or with minimal dilution accompanied by spicy tidbits, leads to strong and quick flare up in the Pitta activity. It causes Uro Daha (Heart burn), Chhardi (Vomiting), Trushna (thirst) etc.

Persons having a Pitta or Pitta Kapha constitution, who are impatient and short-tempered when they indulge in alcohol consumption either strong varieties or in the afternoon, late night or in summer / autumn, after heavy physical workout, on empty stomach lead to intense Pitta accentuation. This again affects liver function badly. The accumulated Pitta results into Bahupitta Kamala (Jaundice) having symptoms such as burning sensation, fever, thirst, yellow stools and urine etc. Avoiding alcohol intake can substantially reduce the intensity of the disease.

Vyadhi Nama : Yakrut Paka / Shopha

Dosha : Pitta, Kapha

Srotodushti : Anna, Rasa, Rakta, Mamsa and Majja vaha srotas

Udbhavasthana : Mahasrotas

Vyaktisthana : Raktavaha, Majjavaha srotas

Avayava : Yakrut

Prakopaka Guna : Ushna, Tikshna, Vikasi and Vyavayi

Pradhana Rasa : Amla, Katu

Srotodushti Prakara : Atipravrutti, Sanga, and Vimargagamana

Antima Parinama : Apatarpanatmaka (Wasting, Atrophy)

Yakrut Shosha

Strong alcoholic beverages made by using inferior quality ingredients like molasses, rotten jaggery etc. consumed with pungent substances like chilies and salts, spices etc. by a Vata constitution person, either in the evening or late night, similarly, strong alcoholic beverages consumed under a peculiar mental state of either fear, grief, after heavy physical work or sexual intercourse leads to vitiation of Vata and Pitta. Strong drinks owing to their dry, light, subtle, Vyavayi and Vikasi attributes cause depletion of body tissues, leading to a state of Shosha. Most affected tissues are Meda, Mamsa and the fluid content of other body constituents. This leads to drying out or wasting of organs. When this Samprapti takes place in the liver initially, it reacts by exhibiting Shotha, which is gradually replaced by Shosha. Sharpness and heat of Pitta in combination with dryness and roughness of Vata leads to drying out the liver. This results in shrinking of liver with rough margins and a hard appearance to touch.

Hepatic Disorders

The combined action of Vata and Pitta leads to depletion of the fluid content of Pitta i.e. mild unctuousness, fluidity and Sarata are depleted this leads to dryness, heat, intensity, roughness of it. This is manifested as pain in abdomen, thirst, tremor and giddiness with the help of Samana Vayu. The enhanced dryness prevents the movement of Pitta from the Raktavaha Srotas i.e. liver. hence the generated Pitta cannot reach the gut but gets mixed in the blood stream. This presents as a chronic medium grade Jaundice, with considerable emaciation and Ojus depletion. The dried out shriveled liver cannot generate enough Pitta to digest food but the vitiated Pitta owing to its intense and hot nature causes internal breakdown of internal lining. These fraying of the internal Kala results in development of ulcerations, which tend to bleed on stimulus like chilies, fast etc. Development of successive Dhatus is also hampered, hence, Rasa gets accumulated and causes abdominal disorders and Shotha. Due to this disturbance, the quantity of Kleda, which has to be generated during this process, is reduced. This causes the reduction in quantity of urine.

Vyadhi Nama : Yakrut Shosha

Dosha : Vata, Pitta

Srotodushti : Anna, Rasa, Rakta, and Mamsa

Udbhavasthana : Mahasrotas

Vyaktisthana : Raktavaha srotas

Avayava : Yakrut

Prakopaka Guna : Tikshna, Ruksha, Ushna, Vikasi and Vyavayi

Pradhana Rasa : Katu

Srotodushti Prakara : Shosha, Siragranthi (Micro, macro nodular liver parenchyma) and Vimargagamana

Antima Parinama : Apatarpanatmaka (Wasting, Atrophy)

Medomaya Yakrut (Fatty Liver)

Lack of exercise, sleeping in daytime, food causing vitiation of Meda Dhatu, excessive consumption of alcohol leads to vitiation of Medovaha Srotasa. Alcohol consumption is directly responsible for Khavaigunya of liver. Madhura, Snigdha, Guru attributes of food taken and lack of exercise vitiate Kapha and Meda. Alcohol, which is less strong, much diluted with water, when consumed by persons having Kapha constitution, in Vasant, Hemant, Shishir seasons, in early age together cause vitiation of Kapha and Pitta. Similarly Medovaha srotas vitiated due to alcohol, leads to excessive accumulation of Meda in the body. Hence, the factors in the Rasa Dhatu responsible for the development of Meda also get accumulated in the liver. Similarly, the Meda accumulated in the body flows along with the Rasa-Rakta, settles in the liver and Raktavaha Sira. This results into Hepatomegaly, increase in mass of the liver, causing heaviness and fatty changes in liver.

Hepatic Disorders

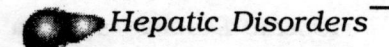

Due to the Madhura, Snigdha attributes, less vitiation of Pitta is occurred and results into Kamala which is of less intensity and prolonged, or the obstructive type of jaundice is seen due to Apachit Meda. The Samprapti caused is Brimhanatmak.

Vyadhi Nama : Medomaya Yakrut (Fatty Liver)

Dosha : Kapha, Pitta

Srotodushti : Rasa, Rakta, and Meda

Udbhavasthana : Mahasrotas

Vyaktisthana : Raktavaha, Medovaha srotas

Avayava : Yakrut

Prakopaka Guna : Mrudu, Madhura, and Amla

Pradhana Rasa : Madhura, Amla

Srotodushti Prakara : Sanga

Antima Parinama : Santarpanatmaka

Sequential Progression Of Alcohol Induced Liver Disorders

Heavy consumption of strong alcoholic beverages &

Vidahi, Pittakara, pungent and spicy food &

Working in sun or near the heat etc.

And

Pitta constitution,

Consuming alcohol in youth or Sharada, Grishma Rutu or late at night

Undiluted alcohol consumption

⇩

Due to Ushna, Tikshna, Amla, Vyavayi, Vikasi properties

⇩

Pitta, Vata vitiation

⇩

Due to Ushna, Tikshna properties, liver tissue gets inflamed

⇩

Due to intense vitiation of Pitta Hepatomegaly occurs

⇩

Vimarga Gamana of Pitta

⇩

Kamala – Ashukari (acute), Teevra Swaroopa (Serious)

Hepatic Disorders

**Heavy consumption of Ruksha and Tikshna (strong) Alcohol &
Diet which helps in vitiating Vata dosha i.e. Ruksha, pungent food &
Stree (excessive sexual indulgence) –Shoka (Grief)-Bhaya (Fear)-Bhara Vahana
karma (heavy physical work)**
And
Vata constitution,
Consuming Alcohol in Grishma, Varsha seasons and late at night
Undiluted alcohol and in old age

⇩

Due to Ruksha, Ushna, Tikshna, Amla, Vyavayi, Vikasi properties

⇩

Vitiation of Vata and Pitta

⇩

Due to Tikshna, Ruksha property tissues of liver are inflamed and Shosha occurs

⇩

Due to Samana Vayu size of liver decreases

⇩

Yakrut Shosha

⇩ ⇩ ⇩

Due to Yakrut Shosha and Ruksha property of Vata obstruction in Vimarga Gamana of Pitta	Vikruta (abnormal) formation of Rakta from Rasa	
⇩	⇩	⇩
Chirakalina Kamala of Madhyama Swarupa	Ghatanatmaka Vruddhi of Rasa	Production of successive Dhatus- badly affected
	⇩	⇩
	Accumulation in Udara	Accumulation in superficial vessels, skin	Production of Kleda
	⇩	⇩	⇩
	Udara disorders	Inflammation (Shotha)	Production of urine decreases
			⇩
			Mutralpata

Hepatic Disorders

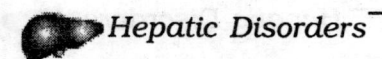

Heavy consumption of Mrudu, Madhura (sweet), Amla Alcohol &
Madhura, Snigdha, Guru food &
Lack of exercise, (Ashrama), sleeping in daytime
And
Kapha constitution,
Consuming Alcohol in Vasanta, Hemanta, Shishira seasons And in Kapha Kala
Much diluted alcohol and in early age

⇩ ⇩

Medovaha Srotodushti   Kapha- Pitta Prakopa
                                                 (Vitiation)

⇩   ⇩

Vikruta Formation of Meda   Madhura, Snigdha properties of
(Yakrutastha Dhatvagnimandya)   vitiation decrease the intensity
                                            of Pitta dosha
⇩   ⇩

Accumulation of Meda in Liver   Intensity of Jaundice decreases

⇩   ⇩

Deerghakalina
Medomaya Yakrut   Accumulation of
(fatty changes)   Apachit Meda
                         ⇩

                        ⇩
Pittavarodha
                     Ruddhapatha Kamala
                     (Obstructive Jaundice)

Hepatic Disorders

So far we have seen the three main types of liver diseases which are observed commonly in practice. The underlying Samprapti also has been describes in textual as well as in a flow chart form. Now we shall see the principle of Chikitsa to manage them. All these conditions are difficult to treat as they exhibit an altered state of the organ either structurally or functionally.

Yakrut Paka

This condition is a result of Pitta and Kapha accentuation. It also has a contribution from the Rasa Rakta, Mamsa, Majja and Anna vaha srotas contamination. This is a condition characterized by presence of Ama. This highly toxic and contaminating substance has to be converted to a harmless form. The principle is Pachana.

Initially in cases of alcohol induced disorder it is advisable to administer a light purgative that will get rid of the vitiated Pitta and Kapha both without damaging the gut. It is called Sramsana. The substances most effectively used are Mrudvika(Vitis Vinifera/ black resins), Aragvadha (Cassia Fistula). Yashtimadhu (G. Glabra), Amalaki (E. Officinalis) and Sita unrefined cane sugar.

After purification to manage the residual doshas, use of Tikta / Bitter and Kashaya / Astringent substances help a lot in the management of this condition.

Arogya Vardhini with Amalaki before meals is useful to improve secretion of Pitta and stimulate Liver function.

Fala Trikadi Quatha is another agent, which improves liver function and reduces Ama formation.

Kalyanaka Ghruta, Dadimadi Ghruta is helpful in combating the irritated dhatus and soothes them by providing vital nourishment. They have a Rasayana effect too, which ensures an uninterrupted Sneha supply to the tissues.

Pravala Panchamruta is an excellent drug in the management of alcohol induced liver disorder. It should be given with Amalaki Khanda Paka.

Kamadudha with Mukta is an excellent drug to combat the sensory involvement like lack of taste, fatigue, delirium, burning, thirst etc.

Sarvanga Abhyanga with Chandana Bala Lakshadi Taila is useful.

Bath with Triphala powder is indicated in case of itching.

Kumari Asava, Balarishta, Rohitakarishta are useful in stimulating the Pitta secretion after the management as Rasayana.

Hepatic Disorders

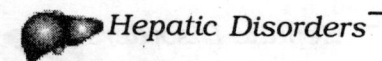

Yakrut Shosha

This is a condition characterized by heightened activity of Vata and Pitta with the unctuousness and fluidity depletion. Here the aim should be to try and replace the depleted Mamsa, Meda, Rasa and Ojus. The Agni is at a low intensity hence not very helpful to combat the condition. Logically the Rasa that would suit the bill perfectly is Madhura. But since it is the heaviest and coldest it cannot be used as it is. Hence Ghee prepared from Pitta Shamaka Rasas like Tikta and Kashaya are used. Use of Guduchi (Tinospora Corifolia) Swarasa to prepare Baffalo Ghee is useful.

Use of Yashtimadhu (G. Glabra) Ksheera Paka to prepare Ghee in the morning in a graded dose is useful to induce regenerative activity.

Mukta Pishti with Yashtimadhu and Gokshura (T. Terrestris) halfway through meal (Samana Kala) helps in restoring the depleted Sneha and Drava from the tissues. Mukta has a decisive role in controlling the Pitta activity at the gut as well as the Dhatu levels. It has a beneficial effect on Ojus and the sensory motor apparatus.

Dhatri Rasayana at Rasayana Kala is helpful in restoring the depleted Mamsa, Meda and Ojus. It also helps restore Agni function.

Suvarna Makshika Bhasma , Pravala Pishti and Lauha Bhasma with Amalaki Khanda Paka at Rasayana Kala are useful.

Drakshasava to stimulate Agni at Samana Kala.

Ashwagandharishta or Balarishta to tone up and build the depleted Mamsa and Meda.

Sarvanga Abhyanga with Ksheera Bala taila in the evening followed by a bath or sponging with Neem (Melia Azadiracta) leaf water is helpful using Black Gram floor and milk paste instead of soap in the morning.

A pack of Dhanvantara Taila on the liver region for 30 mins. In the evening is helpful in restoring the lost Sneha and Drava thus alleviating Shosha.

Suvarna Sutshekahara Rasa with Kushmanda Avaleha at bedtime(Udana Kala) is very effective in CNS symptoms.

Medomaya Yakrut

This is a condition characterized by infiltration of liver by contaminated Meda. Meda, giving rise to enlarged liver having smooth appearance and a firm touch replaces the broken liver cells. Since alcohol has a special affinity to Meda metabolism in the body, we find this phenomenon affecting other organs like heart, kidney too. The principle here is to restore Meda.

Hepatic Disorders

Initially, substances like Sharapunkha (tephrosia purpura), Rohitaka, Nagadanti, Katuka are used.

Tamra Bhasma singly with limejuice is useful in reducing Meda and stimulating liver function.

Loha Bhasma or Mandura Bhasma is indicated in cases of Pandu with Gomutra (cow's urine).

Shilajitvadi Vati with Gold is used as Rasayana.

Vajra kshara or Sharapunkha Kshara with equal parts honey and Ghee at Samana Kala is useful in controlling Meda activity. They also stimulate the Agni, thereby reducing accumulated Ama.

Dr. Vilas Nanal
Saraswati Sadan, Kunthe Chowk, Lakshmi Road, Pune

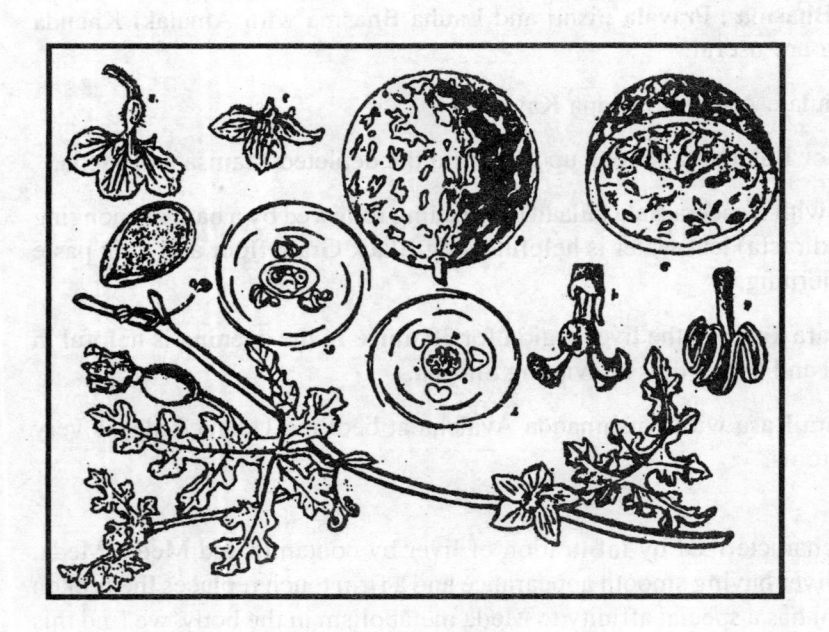

Sanskrit Name : Indravaruni
Latin Name : Citrulus colocynthis

Hepatic Disorders

Comparative Efficay Of Five Indigenous Compound Formulations In Patients Of Acute Viral Hepatitis.

S. V. Dange, P. S. Patki, S. S. Pawar,
S. A. Phadke, D. S. Shrotri

Introduction

Viral hepatitis, a major public health problem throughout the world, occurs in both epidemci and endemic forms in India. Despite rapid advances in modern scientific medicine, there is no specific treatment available for this disease. A number of indigenous agents are claimed to be useful for treatment of liver disorders including viral hepatisi$_2$. We selected five commonly available indigenous compound formulations viz. Arogyavardhini, Hepax, Valiliv, Kamalahar forte and Liv. 52 (See Tables I, II, III, IV and V for composition). In our another study, these agents were found beneficial in a model of hepatocellular jaundice in albino rats. This is the report of comparative efficacy of these agents in patients of acute viral hepatitis.

Patients And Methods

Patients of viral hepatitis, referred to Naidu Hospital, Pune, were included in the study, which extended from June 1985 to June 1987. Two hundred forty eight consecutive adult cases were randomized, after obtaining informed written consent. The diagnosis of acute viral hepatitis was established by history, clinical examination and liver function tests. Patients with history of jaundice for more than 4 weeks before admission, chronic alcohol consumption etc. (See Table VI) were excluded.

Treatment was started within 24 hours after admission. The drugs were given in the form of 2 capsules twice daily for 14 days. Placebo capsules containing 500 mg of dextrose each, were adminstered in the same manner. Patients were asked to take these capsules at least one hour before food. No dietary restrictions were imposed, but patients with severe anorexia and vomiting were treated with intravenous glucose. Likewise bed rest was not imposed. Vit. K was administered to the patients with prothrombin concentrations less than 30% of normal, as estimated by prothrombin time. No other drugs, except B complex vitamins, were allowed.

The following information was obtained before starting treamtnet, twice in first week and then at weekly intervals for next three weeks : state of patient's well being and loss of appetite, presence of any nausea, vomiting, fever, pruritus, rash, joint pains, abdominal discomfort, tiredness, colour of urine, hepatic tenderness and eulargement and some of the liver functions tests (serum bilirubin (normal value < 0.8 mg/dl.)

SGPT (< 25 iu / l), SGOT (< 20 iu / l), alkaline phosphatase (3-13 KAU / dl) and prothrombin concentration (> 60%). Estimations of body weight, hemoglobin, WBC count (Total and differential, serum proteins total (6.3 – 7.9 g / dl), albumin (3.7 – 5.3 g / dl) and globulin (1.8 – 3.6 g / dl) and routine urine examination were done initially and then at the end of four weeks. Hepatitis B surface antigen (HbsAg) was determined at the beginning and at monthly intervals, if positive, by counterimmunoelectrophoresis. The sera were cross checked for SbsAg by RPHA. The clinical features were scored with the help of an arbitary scoring system viz. Absent 0, mild 1, moderate 2 and severe 3. Side effects, likely to be due to the treatment were also recorded. For those patients, who were discharged before the end of four weeks, evaluation was continued on out patients basis. Compliance to therapy was assessed by direct questioning.

Patients were followed up at monthly intervals for a total period of six months from the day of admission. The data were analysed by student's unpaired "t" test, de Jonge's trend analysis and Fisher's exact test.

Results

Two hundred forty eight patients were included in the study. Out of these thirty four patients were excluded from the analysis for reasons mentioned in Table VII.

Thus, 214 patients remained in the trial and received Arogyavardhini (n = 30), Hepax (n = 20), Valiliv (n= 23), Kamalahar Forte (n = 19), Liv. 52 (n = 34) and Placebo (n = 88). The clinical and laboratory details of these patients are summarized in Tables VIII and IX respectively. There was no significant difference in the various groups on entry in the study.

Table X outlines the results of treatment, Treatment with all agents was associated with significanly ($P < 0.05$) less loss in body weight and rapid clinical recovery, as compared to placebo. This was most prominent in patients treated with Arogyavardhini. In drug treated patients, there was significantly ($p < 0.05$) rapid biochemical recovery, as suggested by short time required for 50% decline in serum bilirubin levels and for normalization of SGPT levels. Again this was more marked in those treated with Hepax and Arogyavardhini. By the end of four weeks, 83 to 90 % of patients treated with Arogyavardhini and Hepax had recovered in contrast to 63 to 74 % in those treated by other agents.

The changes in serum levels of bilirubin during the study period of four weeks are shown in Fig. 1. There was a more rapid ($p < 0.05$) decline in the serum bilirubin levels in all drug –

Hepatic Disorders

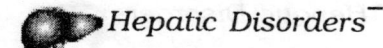

treated patients. It was evident from seventh day of treatment with all agents except Arogyavardhini & Hepax, with which the effect began as early as 4th day. The effects were persistent for a week after stopping treatment. Changes in SGPT levels and in serum levels of alkaline phosphatase were similar to those in serum bilirubin.

There was no significant change in other parameters viz. Serum proteins, SGOT, prothrombin time and clearance of HbsAg etc.

Eight patients from placebo and six patients on drugs had relapse of hepatitis (during fourth (n = 8) and seventh (n = 6) week respectively), from which they recovered uneventfully. No relapse was observed in those treated with Arogyavardhini and Hepax.

Side effects likely to be due to treamtent were recorded in all the groups. These were minor, like diarrhoea, epigastric pain, skin rash etc. and discontinuation of the drug was not required. The incidence of side effects was comparable in all the groups.

During the follow up, 79 patients dropped out from the study at various time intervals., remaining 135 patients (drugs – 82 and placebo – 53) were followed for a period of six months. Seroconversion from HbsAg positivity was noticed in one patient treated with Arogyaardhini and two patients on Hepax, at the end of one month. This was not statistically significant as compared to placebo treatment. Similarly none of the drugs had any significant effect on the incldence of HbsAg carrier state, however the number of cases of hepatitis B in each group was very small.

Discussion

The results show a more rapid clinical as well as biochemical recovery from acute viral hepatitis during treatment with all agents in this study. Although adiminstration of steroids leads to clinical improvement and lowering of serum bilirubin, this is often associated with troublesome side effects and high relapse rate3. Previous studies have demonstrated better clinical improvement in patients of viral hepatitis treated with Liv. 52, 4 Arogyavardhini5 and Stimuliv6. However, the biochemical recovery was unalterd. Besides this, the patient were not followed up to study the effect of drug treatment, if any, on the relapse rate and incidence carrier state in type B hepatitis.

In this study, we have noticed that none of these agents was beneficial in patients of acute viral hepatitis positive for HbsAg. Although the number of patients studies is too small, treatment with Hepax / Arogyavardhini might accelerate the seroconversion in such cases and deserves further study in hepatitis B. The relapse rate and incidence of carrier state were also not modified by any of the preparations studied.

In contrast to this, HbsAg negative patients showed beneficial effects with all treatment, especially with Arogyavardhini and Hepax. The dramatic decrease in total serum bilirubin, evident from 4th day of treatment suggests that these agents might be enhancing bilirubin clearance by stimulating either hepatic or extrahepatic clearance of bilirubin. One of the main ingredients of these preparations viz. Picrorrhiza Kurrooa has been reported to exert such action7. A paniculata and Tuinospora codifalia have been reported to possess hepatoprotective action. 8, 9 There are few reports regarding the pharmacological activity of other ingredients present in these formulations. Hence, it is not possible to comment upon their inclusion. tO our knowledge, this is the first report of comparative efficay of indigenous compound formulations in patients of acute viral hepatits. The results suggests rapid clinical and biochemical recovery with drug treatment in HbsAg negative patients.

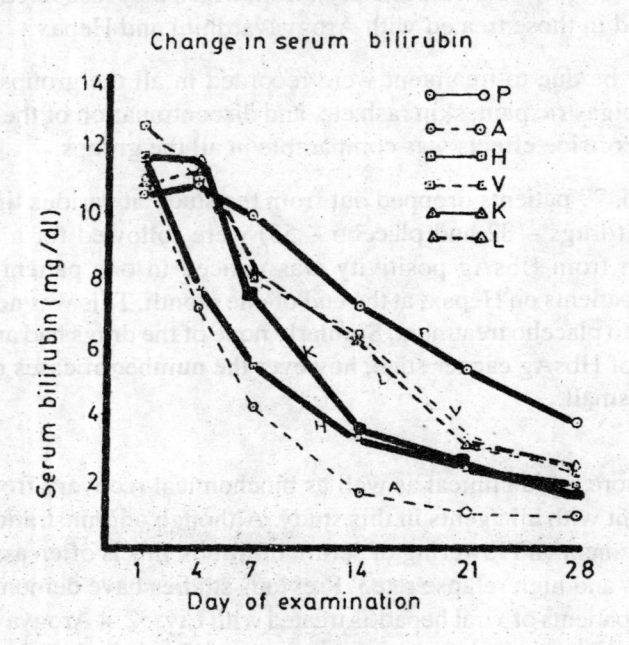

Change in serum bilirubin

The administration of indigenous compound formulations like Arogyavardhini was found beneficial in patients of acute viral hepatitis. There was a rapid clinical and biochemical recovery, most marked in those treated with Arogyavardhini and Hepax. The beneficial effects were restricted to HbsAg negative patients. The relapse rate and incidence of carrier state were not modified, further studies are necessary to determine the role of such agents in patients with severe hepatitis, type B hepatitis population groups pregnant women, old age etc.

Hepatic Disorders

Abstract

Viral hepatitis is a major public health problem in our country. However, as yet, specific treatment is not available. Many indigenous agents are claimed to be neficial, we studied five indigenous compound formulations viz. Arogyavardhini, Hepax, Valiliv, Kamalahar forte and Liv. 52, in 214 patients of acute viral hepatitis admitted to Naidu Hospital, Pune. The patients were randomly accocated to receive either the indigenous compound formulation or placebo. Response to treatment was assessed by regular clinical examination and periodic estimation of liver function tests viz. Serum bilirubin, SGPT, serum alkaline phosphatase etc. Adverse effects, likely to be attributed to drug tretment were recorded and HbsAg status was also assessed. Treatment with all agents, especially Arogyavardhini and Hepax, accelerated clinical and biochemical recovery in HbsAg negative patients.

Table I : Composition of Arogyavardhini

No.	Ingredient	Quantity
1	Mercury	2 mg
2	Sulfur	2 mg
3	Lohabhasma	2 mg
4	Tamrabhasma	2 mg
5	Abhrakbhasma	2 mg
6	Triphala Churna	4 mg
7	Shilajit	6 mg
8	Guggul (Commiphora mukul)	8 mg
9	Chitrakamal churna	8 mg
10	Kutaki churna	36 mg
11	Decoction of A indica	128 mg
Total		200 mg (Approx)

Table II : Composition of Hepax (500 mg)

No.	Ingredient	Quantity
1	P-lumbago zeylanica (Chitraka)	30 mg
2	Picrorrhiza Kurrooa (Kali Kutki)	30 mg
3	Piper Nigrum (Kali Miri)	30 mg
4	Zingiber officinal (Suntha)	30 mg
5	Carbonate of soda (Sajikhar)	30 mg
6	Phyllanthus emblica (Amla)	25 mg
8	Calcium hydroxide (Chuna)	25 mg
9	Pearlash (Papadkhar)	275 mg

Table III : Composition ov valiliv (250 mg)

No.	Ingredient	Quantity
1	Arogyavardhini	60 mg
2	Picrorrhiza Kurrooa	15 mg
3	Termalia chebula	15 mg
4	Eclipta alba	30 mg
5	Solanum nigrum	15 mg
6	Kanthloh bhasma	15 mg
7	Caparis spinosa	15 mg
8	Fumaria parviflora	15 mg
9	Tamarix gallica	10 mg
10	Embelia ribes	15 mg
11	Somnathi tamra	45 mg

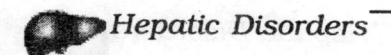

Table IV : Composition of Kamalahar Forte (250)

No.	Ingredient	Quantity
1	Cichoriam intybus	25 mg
2	Solanum nigrum	50 mg
3	Mineral salts	75 mg
4	Mandur bhasma	20 mg
5	Terminalia arjuna	20 mg
6	Achyaranthes aspera	15 mg
7	Tinospora cordifolia	10 mg
8	Tephrosia purpurea	12 mg
9	Boerhavia diffusa	5 mg
10	Emblica officinalis	5 mg
11	Terminalia chebula	3 mg
12	Andrographis paniculata	3 mg
13	Berberis aristata	3 mg
14	Plumbago zeylanica	3 mg

Table V : Composition of Liv. 52 (275 mg)

No.	Ingredient	Quantity
1.	Capparis spinosa	65 mg
2.	Cichorium intybus	65 mg
3.	Solanum nigrum	32 mg
4.	Cassia occidentalis	16 mg
5.	Terminalia arjuna	32 mg
6.	Achillea millefolium	16 mg
7.	Tamarix gallica	16 mg
8.	Mandur Bhasma	33 mg

Table VI : Exclusion Criteria

1. Duration of jaundice > 4 weeks
2. H/o chronic alcoholism
3. H/o Intake of hepatotoxic drugs.
4. Age < 14 yrs., > 50 yrs.
5. Pregancy.
6. Signs of hepatic coma/ precoma.
7. Serum Alkaline Phosphatase > 30 KAU / dl.
8. Associated major illness like diabetes mellitus, renal disease etc.

Table VII : Drop-outs from the study

No.	Reason	Number
1.	Developed coma / precomma	11
2.	Non-compliance with therapy	12
3.	Did not complete 4 weeks observatin period	11
	Total	34

Hepatic Disorders

Table VIII : Clinical Features on Entry

No.	Feature	Arogyavardhini	Hepax	Valiliv	Kamalahar forte	Liv.52	Placebo
1.	Age (years)	28.40±5.60	26.40±7.70	26.60±9.10	30.05±10.94	23.40±8.50	28.11±9.31
2.	Sex (M/F)	17/13	15/6	13/10	12/7	22/12	66/22
3.	Weight (Kg)	46.40±9.32	51.50±10.25	49.70±11.30	52.10±10.25	50.80±10.70	49.06±10.98
4.	Duration of illness (days)	13.23±5.65	11.20±5.03	9.80±4.10	13.10±5.00	10.25±4.25	11.33±4.91
5.	Severity of illness (score)	15.10±4.46	16.25±3.50	16.50±3.70	15.80±4.25	15.45±4.60	14.96±4.54

Table IX Biochemical Profile on Entry

No.	Feature	Arogyavardhini	Hepax	Valiliv	Kamalahar forte	Liv.52	Placebo
1	Serum bilirubin (mg/dl)	11.00±5.91	11.72±6.50	12.50±6.80	11.60±6.80	10.85±6.20	10.49±6.01
2	SGPT (iu/l)	117.18±86.19	125.35±57.67	140.00±60.20	130.52±60.14	130.50±65.20	120.55±74.22
3	Serum Alkaline Phosphoatase (KAU/dl)	16.56±5.75	16.90±6.01	17.30±9.50	16.34±6.10	15.80±8.25	17.37±8.12
4	Serum Proteins (g/dl)						
	Total	6.40±0.72	6.56±0.80	6.90±1.10	6.54±0.87	6.60±0.84	6.81±0.85
	Albumin	4.08±0.36	4.12±0.41	4.40±0.60	4.14±0.44	4.20±0.42	2.53±0.47
	Globulin	2.32±0.40	2.44±0.41	2.50±0.60	2.40±0.44	2.40±0.42	2.59±0.43
5	HbsAg status						
	by CIE (+ve/-)	5/25	6/14	6/17	5/14	8/26	25/63
	By RPHA (+ve/-ve)	10/20	10/20	9/14	8/11	17/20	39/49

Fogires are mean ± SD. No SIgnificant difference between the groups.

Table X : Response to Treatment

No.	Feature	Arogyavardhini (n = 30)	Hepax (n = 20)	Valiliv (n=23)	Kamalahar forte (n=34)	Liv. 52 (n = 34)	Placebo (n = 88)
1	Weight loss (Kg)	1.08±0.23*	1.00±0.86*	1.30±0.90*	1.13±0.89*	1.25±0.95*	2.15+1.10
2	Time for clinical recovery (days)	7.90±3.29**	11.40±6.68*	14.00±7.10*	12.51±6.87*	12.70±7.18*	20.17+9.70
3	Time for 50% fall in serum bilirubin (days)	6.80±2.79	6.47±3.03	7.90±2.40*	8.12±3.90*	8.46±3.54*	15.05±8.70
4	Time for biochemical recovery (days)	120.06±6.29**	23.79±8.28*	21.00±3.90*	25.10±10.55*	36.40±14.10	54.17+9.35
5	No recovered	25 (83.33)*	18 (90)*	16 (69.50)*	12 (63.16)*	25 (73.53)*	39 (55.68)
6	Relapsing hepatitis	-	-	2	1	3	8
7	HbsAg conversion (by one month) per patients followed	1/5	2/6	0/6	0/5	0/8	0/25
8	HbsAg +ve at end of Six months per-patients followed	0/5	0/3	0/6	1/4	3/8	2/14
9	Side effects (No. of patients)	3	3	3	4	3	9

* P<0.05. ** P<0.01, = Compared to Placebo

Hepatic Disorders

Acknowledgements

We are thankful to Vaidya Khadiwale (Hari Parshuram Aushadhalaya, Pune) Shri N. B. Menon (Anglo-French Drug Co. Bombay), Dr. K. C. Mahanto (Khatore Pharmaceuticals, Orissa) and Dr. Suhasini Sharma (Universal Ayurved, Nagpur) for generous supply of drugs. We would also like to acknowledge Dr. Chavan (Superintendent, Naidu Hospital, Pune) for his kind co-operation and our Research Society for financial assistance. Secretarial assistance by Mr. D. H. Gupta, is solicited.

References

1. Chadha M., Sehgal A., Dhorje S. : An overview of viral hepatitis in India. NIV Bulletin 4(2), 1986.

2. Satyavati G. V. : Pharmacology of Medicinal plants and other Natural Products, in : Current Research in Pharmacology in India (1975-82), Eds. P K. Das and B. N. Dhowan, Indian National Science Academy, New Delhi, 1984, pp. 119 – 145.

3. Gregory CM, Kau B. Pen Kempson, R. L., Miller R. : Steroid therapy in severe viral hepatitis, a double blind randomized trial of methyl prednisolone versus placebo. N Engl J. Med. 294 : 681-687, 1976.

4. Sama S. K., Krishnamurthy L. Ramchandran K and Lal K : Efficacy of an indigenous compound preparation (Liv. 52) in Acute Viral Hepatitis. Indian J Med Res. 64 : 738 0 742, 1976.

5. Antarkar D. S., Vaidya A. B., Joshi J. C. at al. : A double blind clinical trial of Arogyavardhini an Ayurvedic drug in acute viral hepatitis. Indian j. Med Res. 72; 588 – 593, 1980.

6. Kadam D. B., Contractor N. S., Nusale G. C. and Mitra P : Effectiveness of an indigenous drug "Stimulive" in viral hepatitis, La Medicine en France, 3-7, 1985.

7. Kumar S., Mishra A., Chaturvedi G. H. : Hepatobiliary response to Picrorrhiza Kurrooa and Eclipta alba in experimental albino rats. J. Res. Edu. Ind. Med. 33-27, 1982.

8. Chaudhary S. K. Indian J. Exp. Biol. 16 : 830, 1978.

9. Rege N., Dahanukar S., Karandikar S. M. : Hepatoprotective effect of Tinospora cordifolia against carbon tetrachloride induced liver damage, Indian Drugs 21 : 544 – 555, 1984.

S. V. Dange , P. S. Patki, S. S. Pawar,
S. A. Phadke, D. S. Shrotri

Effect Of Arogyavardhini – An Indigenous Compound Preparation, On Serum Lipids In Patients Of Acute Viral Hepatitis

S. V. Dange, P. S. Patki, S. S. Pawar, D. S. Shrotri

Viral hepatitis is a major public health problem in our country. Alterations in serum lipid profile have been reported to occur in this disease. Arogyavardhini – an indigenous compound formulation – is widely use in the management of viral hepatitis. This study was designed to assess the effect, if any, of treatment with Arogyavardhini, on serum lipids, in patients of acute viral hepatitis. Fifty five such patients were alternatively allocated to receive either Arogyavardhini (400 mg twice daily X 14 days) or placebo. They were assessed by regular physical examination and estimation of certain laboratory tests on day 1, 3, 7, 14, 21 and 28 of admission. Serum lipid profile was studied initially and at the end of the study. The data were analysed by Student's 't' test. Fifty patients completed the study. Rapid clinical and biochemical recovery was noticed in those treated with Arogyavardhini (n = 26) in contrast to those who received placebo (n = 24). Serum cholesterol (total) and HDL-cholesterol levels were reduced initially in these patients. Treatment with Arogyavardhini resulted in significant ($P < 0.05$) improvement from these changes. The drug was well tolerated. Therefore, it is concluded that treatment with Arogyavardhini is definitely beneficial in patients of acute viral hepatitis and it also has a favorable effect on serum lipid profile in such cases.

Introduction

Viral hepatitis is a major public health problem in our country. Alterations in serum lipid profile in this disease have been reported recently in Indian literature.[1] These abnormalities might play an important role in the pathogenesis of parenchyma liver disease and therapy should aim at their correction, at least temporarily.[2] Arogyavardhini, an indigenous compound preparation, has been reported to beneficial in patients of acute viral hepatitis.[3,4] This study was designed to assess the effect, if any of treatment with Arogyavardhini (Table I) on serum lipids in patients of viral hepatitis.

Hepatic Disorders

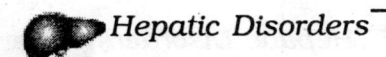

Materials And Methods

A prospective double blind, placebo controlled trial of Arogyavardhini was carried out in patients of viral hepatitis, admitted at Infectious Diseases Hospital, Pune. Fifty five consecutive adult cases were alternately allocated to receive either Arogyavardhini

	Name of ingredient	Quantity
1	Mercury	2 mg
2	Sulfur	2 mg
3	Lohabhasma	2 mg
4	Tamrabhasma	2 mg
5	Abharakbhasma	2 mg
6	Triphala Churna	4 mg
7	Shilajit	6 mg
8	Guggulu (Commiphora mukul)	8 mg
9	Chitrakamul churna	8 mg
10	Kutaki Churna (Picrorrhiza kurrooa)	36 mg
11	Decoction of A. indica	128 mg (Approx.)

or placebo. Informed written consent was obtained. Viral hepatitis was diagnosed on the history, clinical examination and liver function tests. The exclusion criteria are listed in Table 2.

Table 2

Criteria for Exclusion of Patients from the Study

1. Duration of illness < 4 weeks
2. H/o chronic alcohol consumption
3. H/o intake of hepatotoxic drugs
4. Age < 14 years, > 50 years
5. Pregnancy
6. Signs of hepatic coma / precoma
7. Serum ALP > 30 KAU/dl
8. Therapy with immunosuppressants like steroids

Treatment was started within 24 hours after randomization. Arogyavardhini was given in the dose of two tablets (200 mg each) twice daily for 14 days. If necessary, a second course was given. Placebo tablets were administered similarly. The tablets were administered two hours before food. No dietary restrictions were imposed, but patients with severe anorexia and vomiting (nine on Arogyavardhini and seven on placebo) received intravenous glucose. Likewise bed rest was not imposed.

The following information was obtained before starting the treatment, twice in the first week and then at weekly intervals for next three weeks; the state of patient's well being and appetite, the presence of any nausea vomiting, pruritus, abdominal discomfort, rash, joint pains, colour of urine and stools, tiredness, liver tenderness and degree of enlargement, and liver function tests [(serum bilirubin normal value < 1 mg / dl), SALT (<25 IU/l), and serum alkaline phosphatase (SAP) (<13 KAU / dl)]. Estimations of body weight, haemoglobin, total and differential white cell count, serum proteins [total(6.3-7.9 g/dl), albumin (3.7-5.3 g/dl) and globulin (1.8-3.6 g/dl) and routine urine examination were done initially and then at the end of four weeks. Serum lipids viz. Total serum cholesterol (< 250 mg / dl) and HDL cholesterol (< 75 mg / dl) were also estimated at similar intervals by extraction method5 and enzymatic method6 respectively. Hepatitis B surface antigen (HbsAg) was determined at the beginning and at monthly intervals if positive, by counter immuno electrophoresis.

The clinical features were scored with the help of an arbitrary scoring system viz. Absent 0, mild 1, moderate 2, and severe 3. Possible side effects of treatment were also recorded during examination of the patients. For those patients, who were discharged before the end of two weeks treatment period, evaluation was continued as outpatients.

Patients were included in the study from July 1988 to March 1989 and were followed up at monthly intervals for a total period of six months from the day of admission.

The data were analysed by Student's 't' test, de Jonge's trend analysis and Fisher's exact test.

Results

Fifty patients completed the trial. Table 3 shows clinical and laboratory details of the patients in the two groups after decoding of medication. There was no significant difference in the two groups on entry in the study.

Table 3

Clinical and Biochemical Features on Entry

		Placebo (n=24)	Arogyavardhini (n=26)
1	Age (years)	31.56 ± 10.82	28.80 ± 9.72
2	Sex (M : F)	15 : 9	16 : 10
3	Body weight (Kg)	49.80 ± 10.22	46.40 ± 9.32
4	Duration of illness	11.24 ± 5.30	13.20 ± 5.51

Hepatic Disorders

5	Severity of illness (score)	16.30 ± 3.55	15.00 ± 4.56
6	S. Bilirubin (mg / dl)	10.04 ± 3.20	114.26 ± 41.25
7	SALT (iu/l)	106.10 ± 30.45	11.68 ± 3.52
8	SAP (KAU / dl)	17.14 ± 5.80	16.50 ± 4.58
9	S. Proteins (g / dl)		
	Albumin	4.14 ± 0.54	4.05 ± 0.52
	Globulin	2.44 ± 0.32	2.35 ± 0.28
	Total	6.58 ± 0.86	6.40 ± 0.80
10	S. Cholesterol (mg / dl)		
	HDLc	19.38 ± 3.40	18.10 ± 3.16
	Total	6.58 ± 0.86	6.40 ± 0.80
11	HbsAg status		
	(+ ve / - ve)	8/16	10/16

Figures are Mean + S. D.

No significant difference between the groups.

Table 4 outlines the results of treatment. Treatment with Arogyavardhini was associated with significantly ($P < 0.05$) less loss in body weight and rapid clinical recovery as compared to placebo. Biochemical recovery was also rapid as reflected in the shorter time required for 50% decline in serum bilirubin levels and normalization of SALT levels. By the end of 14 days, seven patients recovered from the placebo group in contrast to sixteen from Arogyavardhini group ($P < 0.05$). Serum cholesterol – both total and HDLc were comparably reduced, although in the normal range, in both groups on admission. At the end of four weeks, there was a significant ($P < 0.05$) improvement in these parameters in those treated with Arogyavardhini, as compared to placebo treated patients (Fig. 1) This was also noticed in the ratios viz. HDL Total cholesterol and HDL2/HDL3. The favorable effects of Arogyavardhini on serum proteins (total, albumin and globulin) and clearance of HbsAg were not statistically significant.

Table 4
Response to treatment

		Placebo (n = 24)	Arogyavardhini (n = 26)
1	Weight loss (Kg)	2.70 + 1.20	1.13 + 0.77*
2	Time for clinical recovery (days)	18.04 + 8.94	10.90 + 6.35*

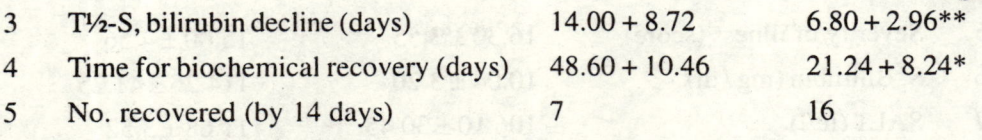

3	T½-S, bilirubin decline (days)	14.00 + 8.72	6.80 + 2.96**
4	Time for biochemical recovery (days)	48.60 + 10.46	21.24 + 8.24*
5	No. recovered (by 14 days)	7	16

Figures are mean + S. D.

* $P < 0.05$, ** $P < 0.01$

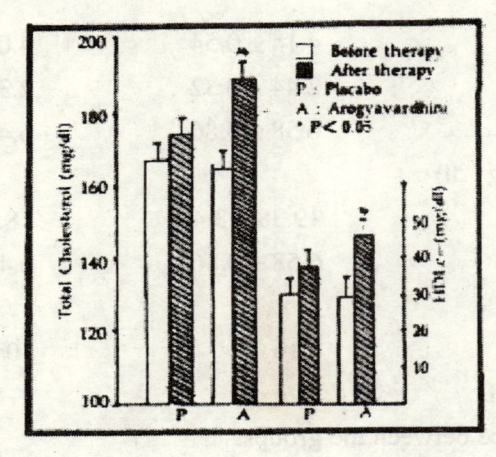

During follow up 32 patients dropped out from the study at various time intervals. Remaining 18 patients (Arogyavardhini 10, placebo 8) were followed for a period of 6 months.

No relapse of hepatitis occurred in any of the patients treated with Arogyavardhini. But 3 patients from placebo group had a relapse without any complication. As the follow up period is 6 months, it is not possible to comment on the development of chronic active hepatitis.

Possible side effects were reported in 3 patients treated with Arogyavardhini (2 had diarrhea, one had pain in abdomen) which did not require discontinuation of medication, while two from the placebo group suffered from pain in epigastrium which could be related to treatment.

Discussion

The results show a more rapid clinical and biochemical recovery from viral hepatitis during treatment with Arogyavardhini. The beneficial effects were also noticed on some serum lipid parameters.

Relief from symptomatology and lowering of serum bilirubin have also been reported with administration of steroids[7] and some other indigenous agents.[8,9] but steroids often produce troublesome side effects and increase the relapse rate. Indigenous agents studied so far did not reduce the time required for biochemical recovery and their effect on relapse rate was not studied. The present study show Arogyavardhini to be better as regard the biochemical activity and early relapse.

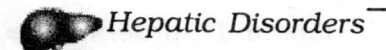

Alterations in plasma lipids and lipoproteins might be responsible for changes in lipid composition of RBC membrane[10] and abnormal permeability to sodium ions. Similar changes occurring in platelets and membranes of other cells could contribute to the general disturbance of cellular function found in patients with severe liver disease.[2] Although it is recommended that therapy should aim correcting these abnormalities at least temporarily, no agent is known to possess such action. Treatment with Arogyavardhini might be promising in this respect, apart from other favorable effects Recently, HDL_C has been reported to be a sensitive parameter of hepatic function in infective hepatitis.[11] Further studies estimating HDL_C at more frequent intervals may be necessary to know, hot treatment with Arogyavardhini affect the same.

The mechanism of action of Arogyavardhini in viral hepatitis is not well know, the lowering of serum bilirubin might be due to stimulation of bile flow [12] induction of microsomal enzymes [13] which have been reported with picrorrhiza kurrooa, main ingredient of Arogyavardhini. Ansari et al[14] have reported the hepatoprotective activity of Kutki, the iridoid glycoside mixture from picrorrhiza kurrooa. Recently, picroliv the active principle of this glycoside mixture was found to protect isolated hepatocytes against thioacetamide induced toxicity (Visen P. K. S. personal communication). These actions may lead to early restoration of depressed lecithin cholesterol acyl transferase activity and thereby correct the altered lipid levels.

To summarize, Arogyavardhini treatment is beneficial in viral hepatitis, as indicated by faster clinical and biochemical recovery, and favorable effects on altered serum lipids. Its effects on severe acute hepatitis, clearance of HbsAs from serum and on chronic liver disorders remain to be investigated.

Acknowledgement

We would like to acknowledge Dr. P. M. Bulakh, Professor of Biochemistry and his staff for extending the co-operation to estimate liver function tests. We are also thankful to Vaidya Khadiwale, Hari Parashuram Aushadhalaya, Pune for generous supply of Arogyavardhini and placebo.

References

1. Vadivelu N., Ramkrishnan S. HDL : total cholesterol and HDL2 : HDL3 cholesterol ratios in liver diseases. Indian J. Med Res. 1986; 83 : 46-52.
2. Mcintyre N. Plasma lipids and lipoproteins in liver disease, Gut 1978; 19 : 526 – 30.
3. Antarkar D. S., Vaidya A. B., Doshi J. C. et al. A double-blind clinical trial of Arogyavardhini – an Ayurvedic drug in acute viral hepatitis. Indian J. Med Res. 1980; 72 : 588-93.
4. Dange S. V., Patki P. S., Pawar S. S., Phadke S. A., Shrotri D. S. Efficacy of Arogyavardhini, an Indigenous Compound Formulation, in Acute Viral Hepatitis. A double – Blind study. Indian Practitioner 1987; 55 : 1063-9.

5. Zak B., Dickenman R. C., White E. G., Burnett H., Chenrey Dj. Rapid estimation of free and total cholesterol. Am J Clin Pathol. 1954; 24 : 1307-15.
6. Wilson D. E., Spiger M. J. A dual precipitation method for quantitative plasma lipoprotein measurement without ultracentrigugation J Lab Clin Med. 1973; 82 : 473-82.
7. Blum A. L., Stutz R., Haemerli U. P. et al. A fortuitously controlled study of steroid therapy in acute viral hepatitis. Am J. Med. 1969; 47 : 82-92.
8. Sama S. K., Krishnamurthy L. Ramchandran K., Lal K. Efficacy of an Indigenous Compound Preparation (Liv. – 52) in Acute Viral Hepatitis – A Double Blind Study. Indian J. Med Res. 1976; 64 : 738-42.
9. Bhandari S. Tak S. K. Indigenous Compound Preparation (Stimuliv) in Childhood Acute Viral Hepatitis. Indian Practitioner 1982; 35 : 487-93.
10. Cooper R. A. Lipids of human red cell membrane : normal composition and variability in disease. Semaine Haematologie. 1970; 7 : 296-322.
11. Nayak S. S., Vasu K. S. Kundaje G. N., Aroor A. R. HDL-cholesterol – A sensitive Parameter of Hepatic Dysfunction in Infective Hepatitis. J. Assoc. Physicians Ind. 1989; 37 : 521-3.
12. Pandey V. N., Chaturvedi G. N. effect of different extracts of kutaki on experimentally induced abnormalities in the liver. Indian J. Med. Res. 1969; 57 : 503-12.
13. Kumar S., Mishra A., Chaturvedi G. H. Hepatobiliary response to Picrorrhiza kurrooa and Eclipta alba in experimental albino rats. J. Res. Edu Ind Med. 1982; 1 : 33-7.
14. Ansari R. A., Aswal B. S., Chander R. et al. Hepatoprotective activity of kutki – the iridoid glycoside mixture of Picrorrhiza kurrooa. Indian J. Med Res. 1988; 87 : 401-4.

S. V. Dange, P. S. Patki, S. S. Pawar, D. S. Shrotri

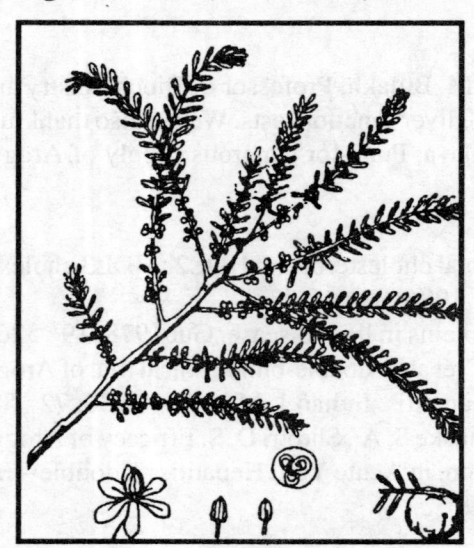

Sanskrit Name : Amalaki
Latin Name : Emblica officinalis

Hepatic Disorders

Role Of Liver In Skin Diseases

Dr. Milind Pendharkar

In Ayurved it is clearly mentioned that pathogenesis of every disease starts from Amashaya. When we go through Nidan & Chikitsa of all diseases; we observe same; up to some extent, but in few diseases we have to think more behind that. Liver is such a vital organ, which has its importance in pathogenesis of such diseases. Through this paper I want to highlight its importance regarding Skin diseases.

In Ayurvedic samhitas Skin diseases are described under title 'Kustha'. All skin diseases are divided in two group, namely Maha & Kshudra Kustha. If we go through pathogenesis of these diseases, it is clearly mentioned that causative factors i.e. dietary & behavioral habits play major role in this context.

Samprapti

वातादयस्त्रयो दुष्टास्त्वग्रक्तं मांसमम्बु च ।
दूषयन्ति स कुष्ठानां सप्तको द्रव्यसंग्रह: ॥

Vatas, Pitta, Kapha, Blood, Mansa, Skin & lymph are basic factors, which get affected in Kustha. Percentage of their affection differs in all types from each other. Tri-dosha, when get vitiated due to causative factors, change their routine action & trough Ras & Rakta they affect Skin. Lymph, Blood & Mansa. Finally we observe symptoms of Kustha.

Treatment

Kustha or skin disease can be treated with Shodhan & Shaman type of treatment. Considering pathogenesis we can judge importance of Shodhan. In Samhitas there is also description about this type of treatment, but in my opinion we can treat only Maha kustha in this way. Considering life style, most of the time we have to plan treatment more with Shaman than Shodhan. In this context our basic Samhitas can't give specific guidelines, that what type of line of treatment we should plan. Other than Nidan parivarjan there is description of many drug combinations for treatment. After clinical experience of few years I can say that, we must think of Liver when we arrange specific line of treatment.

यकृत् प्लिहानौ शोणितजौ ।

Liver & Spleen originate from Blood that is basic assumption of Ayurved. 3 dosha, 7 Dhatus & 3 mala contribute in body constitution. Out of theses, Blood or Rakta is second Dhatu, & it works as Jeevan. The dietary components that we eat get digested in Amashaya & Pachak ras get prepared. All 7 Dhatus get nourished with this one by one. If Agni is not working properly all Dhatus will not be nourished properly, which causes improper formation of Mala also. As I said earlier, causative factors vitiate Tri-dosha, & finally all these things collectively do Srotorodha in Liver. Due to all these changes, function of Jeevan can't take place ideally, which finally affects Skin, Lymph, Blood & Mansa, thus we describe pathogenesis of Kustha.

If we consider Tri-dosha, each Dosha is of 5 different types. Pitta also is of 5 different types. Out of these Pachak & Ranjak pitta are related with Liver. Pachak pitta digests food & Ranjak pitta helps in nourishment of Dhatu like, Rakta, Mansa, and Meda etc. If digestion is not proper Skin & other organs can loose their Vyadhi-kshamatva or Immunity. When we treat any case of skin disease we must consider above said points before prescribing particular line of treatment.

Discussion

As I said skin diseases are treated with San Shodhan & San Shaman type of treatment. In this paper I have discussed Shaman. For this type of treatment there are various drugs & all these can be given in various ways i.e. in the form of Swaras, Quath (Decoction), Asav, Arista, Bhasmas, Rasoushadhi, etc. which act systemically. If we go through all these drugs we observe drugs mainly titled as Kusthaghana. Here I shall discuss some important medicines to express my view.

Karanj :- (Pongamia pinnata) – With its Katu & Tikta properties it is good digestive, carminative & blood purifier. Due to Tikshana it acts as wormicidal & liver stimulant with good collective action on skin.

Nimb :- (Azadirachta indica) – Due to Tikta & Kashaya it is wormicidal, blood purifier, liver stimulant with Kushthaghna property.

Khadir :- (Acasia catechu) – It is anti inflammatory, blood purifier, having coagulation property due to Tikta & Kashaya property. It is also Kushthaghana & Kandughna (minimizes itching).

Haridra :- (Curcuma longa – It is blood purifier, enhances skin color, Kandughna, Wormicidal, having action as liver stimulant.

Chakramarda : (Cassia tora) – With Katu & Ushna it acts as wormicidal, Kushthaghna & liver stimulant.

Hepatic Disorders

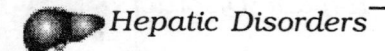

Manjistha – (Rubia Cordifolia) – It is blood purifier, wormicidal, kusthaghna, digestive, liver stimulant.

Sariva – (Hemidesmus indicus) – Anti inflammatory, blood purifier, liver stimulant, special action in pittaj skin diseases.

Arogya-vardhini : Main contents are Kajjali, Loh, Abhrak, and Tamra. All these have good action on liver. Its main ingredient Katuki has good liver stimulant action.

Gandhak rasayan : In this pure Gandhak get processed in shunthi, triphala, guduchi, maka etc. This medicine also shows good action as kusthaghna & liver stimulant.

Kushtha – kuthar ras : Kajjali, Loh, Tamra, Abhrak, Shilajatu, are main metallic powders i. e. bhasmas which has effective action on liver diseases. Karanj seeds are it's main ingredient of which action is discussed previously.

Swayambhuv guggul : Guggul, Bakuchi, Karanj, Haridra, Nimb are main ingredients. All these are good liver stimulant & kusthaghna.

All above said medicines alone or in combination are widely used in skin diseases. Kumari asav, Mahamanjisthadi quath, Sarivadyasav, Vidangarista like asav preparations are also commonly used. In all these, main ingredients also have main action as **Kusthaghna & Liver stimulant**.

In Ayurved treat the disease & plan to avoid relapse is basic view to treat any disease. To avoid relapse immunity of individual is very important. In context with skin disease this management is most important. In skin disease during pathogenesis vitiated dosha become tiryak gami, hence though we observe earlier symptomatic relief relapse is also common. For this we have to treat these patients for long period & to enhance the immunity we have to give Liver stimulant with which nourishment for all Dhatus will be proper. Another point to be highlighted that; along with Shodhan one must give Shaman treatment & medicines for local application, because collective action gives good results.

Conclusion

In Modern science management of skin disorders, skin is considered as a single organ, hence chances of relapse is more; on the other hand along with skin treating liver gives long lasting & enthusiastic results. This is more perspective view in the treatment of skin diseases.

Dr. Milind Pendharkar B.A.M.S., F.I.I.M.,
Ashwini Clinic, 7 Mangalwar Peth, Karad

Hepatic Disorders

33. A Proposed Hepato – Immuno Modulating Drug Regimen For Hepatitis.

Dr. M. V. Acharya.
Dr. Parveen Bansal.

Hepatitis is one of the most common acute liver disorder which is often followed by chronic liver disease such as cirrhosis, hepatic encephalitis and fulminent hepatic failure with grave prognosis and jaundice is the main presenting symptom of all liver disorder including hepatitis of various orgins. The cause of hepatitis according to modern medicine may either be infectious (virus and others) or drugs and chemicals which are directly responsible for the damage of liver cells.

According to recent statistical survey, there are estimated 43 millions (4.3 crore) HBV carriers in our country (4.2%) which represent 10% of the total world HBV pool (second only to China). Out of these 10% are positive for HBV Ag which represent highly infectious and rapidly multiplying virus. About 25% of HBV positive persons get liver disease in life time. HBV is more infectious and dangerous than that of HIV virus because in later condition the patient can survive for years on comparison to months in former. The only and major positive point of HBV is that, safe and effective vaccine is available for it. Till today about 90 countries in the world are practising universal immunization in all newborns but unfortunately no serious attempts have been made in our country.

Ayurveda being more fundamental to its concepts does not describe the micro-organisms like virus bacteria etc., as a potent cause but admitting their existence describe them as an accessory or secondary cause for the disease. If we look into the etiological factors, the provocation of Pitta is mainly responsible for the occurrence. The triggering factor is the pandu which can proceed the disease. As far as the treatment of this disease is concerned still no rational therapy has been documented to treat this disease by of modern medicine but as far as Ayurvedic literature is concerned, it has got a big place which is well known all over the world. Keeping this view in mind, authors have tried to compile a list of herbal drugs that can be administered in hepatits patients. The drug regimen has been prepared based on the

Hepatic Disorders

documented biochemical and pharmacological actions of the known herbs. These herbs include (1) Aegle marmelos (Bilva) (2) Andrographis paniculata (Kiratatikta) (3) Bacopa monnieir (Jala Brahmi) (4) Citrullus lanthus (Indravaruni) (5) Eclipta alba (Bhringaraja) (6) Phyllanthus asperulatus (Bhumyemalaki) (7) Piper longum (Pippali) (8) Pichroza curroa (Katuki) (9) Plumbage zeylanica (Chitramula) (10) Sphaeramthus indicus (Sravani/mundi) (11) Tephrosia purpurea (sharapunkha). Authors feel that the combination of all these herbs may give rise to a potent drug effective for hepatitis. The detailed biochemical and pharmacological actions will be discussed in full paper.

Dr. Middela Venugopal Acharya
Central Research Institute (Ayu), Moti Bagh, Road, Patiala – 147 001
Tel : 0175 – 212393 (O), 212348 (R), Fax : 0175 – 212393

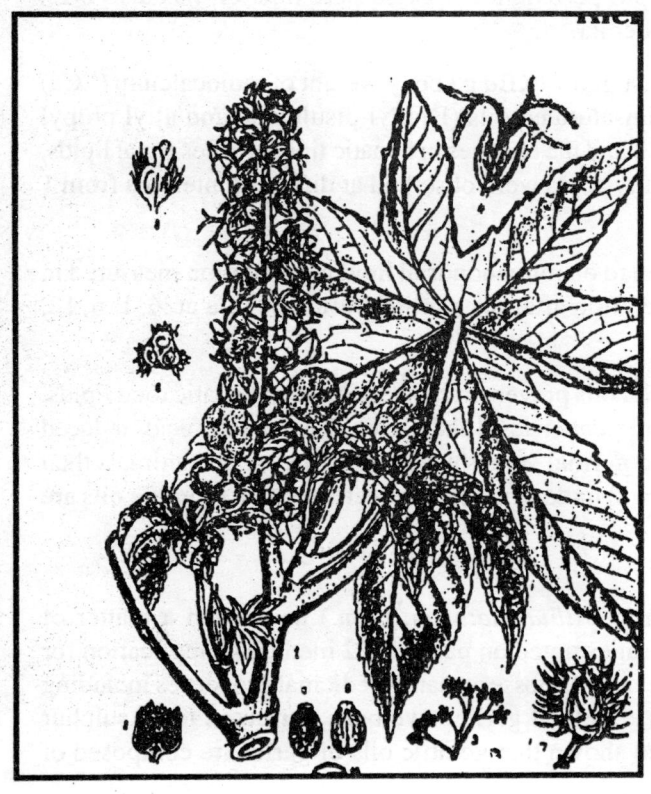

Sanskrit Name : Erand
Latin Name : Ricinus communis

Hepatic Disorders and Antioxidants: Mechanistic Aspects of Oxidative Injury and its Prevention by Garlic (*Allium sativum, Linn.*) unsaturated oils

Navneet Kumar Gupta

Free radicals have been implicated as contributing factor to the development of chronic diseases including hepatic disorders. Ionizing radiation initiate free radical reactions within the cells as evident by induction of lipid peroxidation. Lipid peroxidation has also been demonstrated in experimental hyperlipidemia.

Adult Swiss albino mice were administered 74KBq g^{-1} body weight of radiocalcium (^{45}Ca) in the presence and absence of garlic unsaturated oils (Diallyl disulphide and allyl propyl disulphide 100mg kg^{-1} body weight day^{-1}) and the changes in hepatic lipid profiles (total lipids, triglycerides, phospholipids and free fatty acids were observed at different intervals from 1 to 14 days post treatment.

Also, the effect of garlic oils was studied on mitochondrial lipid peroxidation measured in terms of malanoaldehyde (MDA) generation after the administration of ^{45}Ca at ½, 1, 6, 12, 24 and 48 h post treatment.

The results obtained indicate that garlic oils prevented rapid increase in hepatic total lipids, triglycerides, phospholipids, and lipid peroxidation level and decrease in free fatty acids induced by radio calcium and the values reached normal values earlier in garlic treated animals than in irradiated group. Possible mechanism(s) underlying the protective action of garlic oils are reported.

Introdution

The purported health effects of garlic (*Allium sativum*, Linn.) have been a matter of record since 1500 BC, when Egyptian sages noted on papyrus 22 medicinal application for the smelly bulb. Besides its culinary use, its oils possess many medicinal properties including hypolipidemic action. The therapeutic effects of garlic have been attributed to its sulphur compounds (Temple, 1962). It has been shown that volatile oils of garlic are composed of

Hepatic Disorders

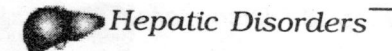

allyl propyl disulphide and diallyl disulphide (Saghir et al., 1964).

With an increasing interest in the role of food to prevent disease and promote good health, garlic has its adherents who are often different than those who find it aromatic and pleasing to palate. There are aims of garlic's efficacy to improve complexion, to cure cancer, impotency, leprosy, tuberculosis, bad blood, hearth diseases (Jain and Apitz-Castro, 1993).

It has repeatedly been observed that irradiation of animals results in increased hepatic lipid accumulation, the increase mainly due to triglycerides build up (Skalka, 1958; Wooles, 1967; De and Aiyar, 1978; Aiyar and De, 1978 and Gupta, 1984). Hyperlipidemia is a high risk factor in heart diseases (Carlson and Bottiger, 1972 and Alprink, 1974) and it has been found that the incidence of heart diseases is low in countries where garlic is widely used, the hypolipidemic action of garlic are pertinent in this context.

Oxidation and production of free radicals are an integral part of mammalian metabolism. Oxygen is the ultimate electron acceptor in a closely linked electron flow system that produces energy in the form of adenosine triphosphate (ATP). Under certain conditions, the electron flow may become uncoupled, leading to the production of free radicals, which are molecules with unpaired electrons and thus very reactive. Examples of free radicals include superoxide (O_2^0), hydroxyl (OH^0), peroxyl (RO_2^0), alcoxyl (RO^0), oxides of nitrogen (NO^0, NO_2^0) and thiyl (RS^0). In addition, free radial reactions may be induced by reactive oxygen containing species (ROS) generated in biological systems. Examples of ROS include singlet oxygen ($^1O_2$), hydrogen peroxide (H_2O_2) (Halliwell et al., 1995, Thomas, 1995). At high concentrations, however, free radicals react with non radicals and can initiate adverse chain reactions such as lipid peroxidation. They also damage other important molecules including proteins, DNA and carbohydrates.

Free radicals have been implicated as contributing factors to aging(Cutler, 1991) and development of chronic diseases including heart disease and cancer (Halliwell et al., 1995; Thomas, 1995; Halliwell et al., 1992 and Papas, 1996). Superoxide radicals (O_2^-) and hydrogen peroxide (H_2O_2) are generated during irradiation and in turn are converted to hydroxyl free radical (OH^0). The hydrogen atom in unsaturated fatty acids can be abstracted by OH radical following the formation of lipid alkyl radical (R^0), which initiates the chain reaction of lipid peroxidation in an aerobic system (Releigh et al., 1977; and Yukawa and Nakazawa, 1980).

Lipid peroxidation alters the membrane fluidity and causes cell degradation, affecting the biological defense mechanisms. Lipid peroxidation is considered to be an important effect of ionizing radiation. Radiation-induced lipid peroxidation has been reported to be caused by super-oxide radicals (O_2^-) (Petkau and Chelack, 1976). However, later studies confirmed that hydroxyl radicals (OH^0) is the most active species involved in radiation peroxidation (Purohit et al., 1980 and Helzer et al., 1980). Lipid peroxidation has been demonstrated in experimental hyperlipidemia (Castro *et al.*, 1974; Yesuda *et al.*, 1980 and Rathi *et al.*, 1984). The present investigation was undertaken to study the protective effect of garlic unsaturated oils in reducing radiation-induced lipid peroxidation and hyperlipidemia in the liver of Swiss albino mice exposed to radiocalcium internal beta irradiation and the possible mechanisms(s) underlying such effects with reference to their proposed antioxidant and free radical scavenging properties are reported.

Materials and methods

Allyl propyl disulphide (C_3H_5-S-S-C_3H_7) and diallyl disulphide (C_3H_5-S-S-C_3H_5) the two unsaturated, volatile oils of garlic were extracted from raw cloves which were sliced, crushed and soaked in diethyl ether for 48 hours as per the method of Sodimu *et al.* (1948) and prepared for experimental use by the modified method of Adamu *et al.* (1982).

Adult male Swiss albino mice of 6-8 weeks with an average weight of 25±2 g were divided into two groups and each group was further divided into two sub-groups having 30 animals in the first sub-group (control) and 90 animals in the second sub group for irradiation (first group) and garlic oils +irradiation (second group). Animals of first group (second sub-group) were injected (ip) 74 KBq g^{-1} body weight of ^{45}Ca (obtained from Bhabha Atomic Research centre, Bombay, in the form of calcium chloride in dilute hydrochloric acid, sp. activity 0.66 GBq g^{-1} of calcium), while animals of group second (second sub-group) were given garlic oils (100 mg Kg^{-1} body weight day^{-1}) as a saline suspension through a stomach tube 2-4 hr before ^{45}Ca injection on the first day and then through out the period of experimentation. Six to ten animals from each group were sacrificed at the intervals of 1, 3, 5, 7 and 14 days post treatment. Liver was excised, blotted dry and processed for biochemical estimation of total lipids (Folch *et al.*, 1957). triglycerides (Amenta, 1964), phospholipids (Silversmit and Davis, 1950) and free fatty acids (Natelson, 1971).

To study lipid peroxidation, animals from both groups were anaesthesized by administration of an overdose of diethyl ether anaesthesia and were killed at ½, 1, 6, 12, 24 and 48 h post treatment. The livers of the animals were perfused with isotonic saline, removed and weighed. A 10% homogenate was prepared in 0.2 m Tris-HCl buffer (pH 7.4). The lipid peroxidation was estimated as per the method of Konings and Drijver (1979).

Results

Animals given either garlic oil or control (normal) did not show any significant change in total lipids (TL), triglycerides (TG), phospholipids (PL) and free fatty acids (FFA) in the liver of mice.

The total lipids content showed a continuous increase from day 1 with a maximum value observed on day 5 post-treatment ($P<0.01$) after ^{45}Ca administration. From day 7, a decline in TL content was observed and near normal values observed on day 14. Triglycerides content also showed a similar trend with maximum value observed on day 5 ($P<0.01$) after

Hepatic Disorders

^{45}Ca injection. Phospholipids content increased upto day 3 (P<0.01). Near control values for TG and PL were attained by day 14 (Fig. 1.1 to 1.3). FFA content showed a continuous decline from day 1 with minimum values observed on day 5 (P<0.01). From day 7, an increase in FFA was discernible and control values were seen on day 14 (Fig. 1.4). In animals of second sub-group of group second, although increase in TL (P<0.05), TG (P<0.05), PL (P<0.05) and decrease in FFA (P<0.05) was evident, yet these values were significantly below those observed for ^{45}Ca group (second subgroup, first group) for TL, TG, PL and higher for FFA. Near control or control values were also seen earlier i.e. on day 7 post-treatment in this group (Fig. 1.1 to 1.4).

The effect of garlic oils on mice mitochondrial lipid peroxidation was measured in terms of malanoaldehyde (MDA) generation after the administration of radiocalcium (^{45}Ca) at ½, 1, 6, 12, 24, 48 h post treatment. The lipid peroxidation level increased significantly from ½ h and reached a peak at 6 h post treatment (P<0.01) and gradually declined thereafter. A decrease in the lipid peroxidation level was observed at 12 h which was approximately 38% less than preceding sampling time. However, lipid peroxidation did not attain normal level even at 48 h post treatments (Fig. 1.5).

In the garlic oil + ^{45}Ca group a significant increase in lipid peroxidation was observed at different intervals, yet it was 27.8%, 29.8%, 43.1%, 28.5%, 27% and 28.3% lower for ½, 1, 6, 12, 24 and 48 h post treatment respectively compared to the concurrent irradiated control (Fig. 1.5).

Discussion

The present study indicated that the administration of ^{45}Ca results in an increase in total lipids, triglycerides and phospholipids contents in the liver of mice. These results are consistent with those of Skalka (1958), Gupta (1984) and others (Wooles, 1967; De and Aiyar, 1978; and Aiyar and De, 1978). An increase in TL content indicates the initiation of lipogenesis including sterols. The biosynthesis of fatty acids requires reducing power in the form of NADPH to reduce double bonds of intermediates in the process and this function is especially prominent in carrying out the biosynthesis of fatty acids and sterols from small precursors. The NADPH required for reductive steps in FA biosynthesis is formed by the reactions of pentose phosphate pathway, especially the activity of G6PDH which is significantly high in ^{45}Ca administered animals as reported earlier (Gupta, 1990). Also, slowing down of the Krebs cycle (Gupta, 1990) would lead to formation and efflux of citrate from mitochondria, which in turn would favour fatty acid synthesis, since substrate availability would increase (Baynen et al., 1980).

Phospholipids participate in the formation of structural elements mainly membranes within the cells throughout the body (Guyton, 1981). It is reasonable to conclude that much of PL content synthesised by hepatic cells be used for the reconstruction of membranes of cellular and sub-cellular membrane organelles which get damaged by internal irradiation.

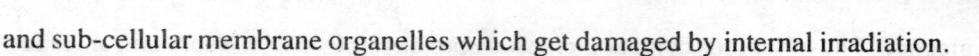

The presence of low levels of FFA in liver suggest that they are being utilized for metabolism. The mobilization of FFA generally occurs in two ways. FFA may enter into lipogensis through esterification and/or they may be reduced to acetyl coenzyme-A to undergo ß-oxidation. However, decreased activity of succinic dehydrogenase (an index to oxidative metabolism) clearly indicates that decrease in FFA levels is due to increased lipogenesis and hence increase in TL, TG and PL and not due to their oxidation.

The observed lipid reducing action of oils indicates the potential medicinal value of garlic. The organic disulphides found in the two oils are good acceptors of hydrogen and their biological actions may be ascribed partly to their reactions with thiol group substances and partly to that with NADPH. The active principles of garlic, viz. allyl propyl disulphide and diallyl disulphide are supposed to be metabolised in the liver utilizing NADPH (Black, 1962; and Kolthoff et al., 1955).

$$C_3H_5\text{-S-S-}C_3H_5 + NADPH + H^+ \quad 2C_3H_5SH + NADP^+$$

$$C_3H_5\text{-S-S-}C_3H_7 + NADPH + H^+ \quad C_3H_5\text{-SH} + C_3H_7SH + NADP^+$$

Thus, the availability of NADPH for FA synthesis will be decreased by the hepatic metabolism of garlic principles. It is established that organic disulphides can inactivate thiol group substances as a result of thiol-disul;phide exchange reactions (Crawhall and Watts, 1968 and Augusti, 1977). As such reaction can inactivate thiol group enzymes like HMG COA reductase and fatty acid synthetase (Gilbert and Stewart, 1981) by exchange reactions of -SH groups of enzymes forming mixed disulphide or intra molecular protein disulphides and also oxidise NADPH and all these are essential for lipid biosynthesis.

$$O\text{-SH} + C_3H_5\text{-S-S-}C_3H_5 \text{ (or } H_7) \quad O\text{-S-S-}C_3H_5 + C_3H_5 \text{ (or } H_7)SH.$$

Thus, administration of garlic oils could have reduced lipid synthesis in the liver of mice exposed to ^{45}Ca internal irradiation and thus responsible for the hypolipidemic action in the present study.

Lipid peroxidation induced by radiation is known to be due to the attack of free radicals on the fatty acid component of membrane lipids (Releigh et al., 1977, Wills and Wilkinson, 1970). Mitochondrial membranes contain high percentage of polyunsaturated fatty acids and are, therefore, susceptible to free radical attack (Bindoli, 1988). Damage to mitochondrial structure and enhanced lipid peroxidation by ionizing radiation has been reported (Kerognou et al., 1981, Yukawa et al., 1985).

The present study indicates that the administration of ^{45}Ca results in an increase in lipid peroxidation (measured as nMol MDA/mg protein) in the liver of mice. These results are in good agreement with earlier findings (Christophersen, 1966; 1968; Ayene *et al.*, 1988; Tretter *et al.*, 1990). Several investigators reported that lipid peroxidation will start as soon as the supply of endogenous reduced glutathione (GSH) is exhausted and that addition of GSH promptly stops the process further (Christophersen, 1966; 1968). A decrease in lipid peroxidation was observed by Ayene *et al.* (1988), in mice erythrocytes treated with MPG before irradiation. Also, GSH and WR-1065 were found to be effective inhibitors of lipid peroxidation by Tretter *et al.* (1990).

In actively metabolising cells, there is considerable water besides the target molecules (DNA, membranes etc.) denoted by RH_2. The 'direct' and 'indirect' actions of radiation would initiate radiation chemical events as follows:

$$H_2O \longrightarrow H^{\cdot} + OH^{\cdot} + e^-_{aq} \quad (i)$$

$$RH_2 \longrightarrow RH^{\cdot}, H^{\cdot}, e^- \text{ (trapped)} \quad (ii)$$

Since O_2 is present in actively metabolising cells, it reacts with reducing species as:

$$H^{\cdot} + O_2 \longrightarrow HO^{\cdot}_2 \quad (iii)$$

$$e^-_{aq} + O_2 \longrightarrow O^{\cdot-}_2 \quad (iv)$$

$$RH^{\cdot} + O_2 \longrightarrow (RH\ O^{\cdot}_2) \quad (v)$$
$$\text{(damaged target molecule)}$$

$$HO^{\cdot}_2 + HO^{\cdot}_2 \longrightarrow H_2O_2 + O_2 \quad (vi)$$

$$H^0 + H_2O_2 \longrightarrow H_2O + OH^{\cdot} \quad (vii)$$

$$OH^{\cdot} + OH^{\cdot} \longrightarrow H_2O_2 \quad (viii)$$

The other pathway of damage to target molecule (RH_2) could be owing to sequential attack by $OH^{\cdot}$ and H_2O_2 as follows:

$$RH_2 + OH^{\cdot} \longrightarrow RH^{\cdot} + H_2O \quad (ix)$$

$$RH^{\cdot} + H_2O_2 \longrightarrow R^{\cdot} + OH^{\cdot} + OH^- + H^{\cdot} \quad (x)$$

From equation (vi) and (viii) it can be seen that hydroxyperoxyl radical ($HO^{\cdot}_2$) and hydroxyl radical ($OH^{\cdot}$) react to yield H_2O_2

$$2H_2O_2 \longrightarrow 2H_2O + O_2 \quad (xi)$$

Since radiation decreases catalase activity (Caldarera *et al.*, 1966; Kergonou *et al.*, 1981), H_2O_2 accumulation should increase. It is established that H_2O_2 inhibits SOD activity (Hodgson and Fridovich, 1975), which may result in increased concentration of Superoxide radical and hence responsible for radiation induced lipid peroxidation. The role of superoxide radials (Petkau and Chelak, 1976) and OH· (Purohit *et al.*, 1980; and Helzer *et al.*, 1980) in lipid peroxidatioin has been confirmed.

Diallyl disulphide and allyl propyl disulphide the volatile oils of garlic can readily accept electrons (e^-aq) which give rise to radical anion and thiyl radicals (Kosower and Kosower, 1976).

$$C_3H_5\text{-S-S-}C_3H_5 + e^-\text{ aq} \longrightarrow C_3H_5\text{-S-S}^{\cdot-}\text{-}C_3H_5 \qquad \text{(xii)}$$

$$C_3H_5\text{-S-S-}C_3H_7 + e^-\text{ aq} \longrightarrow C_3H_5\text{-S-S}^{\cdot-}\text{-}C_3H_7 \qquad \text{(xiii)}$$

$$C_3H_5\text{-S-S}^{\cdot-}\text{-}C_3H_5 \longrightarrow C_3H_5S^- + C_3H_5S^\cdot \qquad \text{(xiv)}$$
$$\text{Radical} \quad \text{thiyl}$$
$$\text{anion} \quad \text{radical}$$

$$C_3H_5\text{-S-S}^{\cdot-}\text{-}C_3H_7 \longrightarrow C_3H_5S^- + C_3H_7S^\cdot \qquad \text{(xv)}$$

The thiyl radicals thus produced react with superoxide radicals as follows:

$$2C_3H_5S^\cdot + 2O^{\cdot-}_2 \longrightarrow C_3H_5\text{-S-S-}C_3H_5 + 2O_2 \qquad \text{(xvi)}$$

The reactions (xii) and (xiii) could possibly diminish the scope for harmful reactions of electrons with O_2 (reaction iv) to result in increased formation of oxidizing species. Further $C_3H_5S^\cdot$ can react also with O_2^- as follows:

$$2C_3H_5S^\cdot + 2O^{\cdot-}_2 \longrightarrow C_3H_5\text{-S-S-}C_3H_5 + 2O_2 \qquad \text{(xvii)}$$

Since $O^{\cdot-}_2$ are responsible for radiation-induced lipid peroxidation, this reaction is possibly protective. Further, the scavenging of OH by C_3H_5 SH or C_3H_7 SH, produced as a result of the oxidative action of garlic oils on NADPH (Black, 1962; and Kolthoff *et al.*, 1955) as shown below:

$$C_3H_5\text{-S-S-}C_3H_5 + NADPH + H^+ \longrightarrow 2C_3H_5SH + NADP^+ \qquad \text{(xviii)}$$

$$C_3H_5\text{-S-S-}C_3H_7 + NADPH + H^+ \longrightarrow C_3H_5SH + C_3H_7SH + NADP^+ \qquad \text{(xix)}$$

$$C_3H_5SH + OH^\cdot \longrightarrow C_3H_5S^\cdot + H_2O \qquad \text{(xx)}$$

$$C_3H_7SH + OH^\cdot \longrightarrow C_3H_7S^\cdot + H_2O \qquad \text{(xxi)}$$

could by itself be protective as the magnitude of $OH^\cdot$ - mediated damage to target molecule (RH_2) (reaction ix and x) would be greatly diminished. Production of H_2O_2 by recombination among $OH^\cdot$ (reaction viii) would also be reduced. In addition, disulphides could also render $HO^\cdot_2$ harmless as shown below:

$$C_3H_5\text{-S-S-}C_3H_5 + HO^\cdot_2 \longrightarrow 2\,C_3H_5S^\cdot + HO^-_2 \qquad \text{(xxii)}$$

$C_3H_5S^\cdot$ (thiyl radical) resulting from a number of different pathways (reactions xiv, xv, xx, xxi, xxii) can react with oxygen as follows:

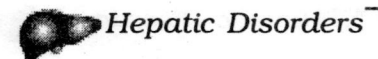

$$C_3H_5S^\cdot + O_2 \longrightarrow C_3H_5SO_2^\cdot \qquad \text{(xxiii)}$$

The overall effect would be a reduction in the availability of O_2 for deleterious reactions.

Reconstitution of target radicals ($RHO_2^\cdot$) can be achieved by a reductive H – transfer reaction.

$$C_3H_5SH + RHO_2^\cdot \longrightarrow RH_2 + C_3H_5S^\cdot + O_2 \qquad \text{(xxiv)}$$
(Restoration)

$$C_3H_5SH + RH^\cdot \longrightarrow RH_2 + C_3H_5S^\cdot \qquad \text{(xxv)}$$
(Restoration)

With regard to thiyl radicals ($C_3H_5S^\cdot$ or $C_3H_7S^\cdot$), it appears unlikely that, in irradiated cells, they might effectively contribute to the inactivation of critical molecules, because in that case thiol depletion should protect oxically irradiated cells and not the other way around, as observed in many cases. It is rather suggested that the ability of thiyl radicals to reversibly react with O_2 can be the key of their role. In fact, it seems reasonable to postulate that the reaction of $C_3H_5S^\cdot$ with oxygen might be in competition with any other oxygen – radical reaction, and being quite fast, it might effectively reduce the amount of O_2 available for damage fixation.

GSH provides a natural defence against ROS and free radicals generated in the cells (Ball, 1966). It has been shown that GSH is markedly oxidised to GSSG during detoxification of radiation induced toxins, such as free radicals, and/or the repair of critically damaged cell structures. GSH can engage in one electron reactions with potentially harmful radicals by hydrogen atom donation, thus forming the relatively stable thiyl radical and ultimately GSSG (Kosower and Kosower, 1976). The ratio between GSSG/GSH, which is a good indicator of oxidative stress is known to increase following radiation exposure. A perturbation in GSSG/GSH ratio could lead to increased lipid peroxidation as seen in the present study.

GSH an be generated from GSSG as shown below:

$$2C_3H_5SH + GSSG \longrightarrow 2C_3H_5S^\cdot + 2GSH \qquad \text{(xxvi)}$$

Thus, elevation of GSH level by garlic oils can play a protective role by disposing of ROS and free radicals. Also, thiyl radicals ($C_3H_5S^\cdot$) can react with oxygen (reaction xxiii) thus reducing the amount of O_2 available for damage fixation and also decreasing/inhibiting formation of superoxide radicals, which are responsible for radiation induced lipid peroxidation.

Therefore, it is reasonable to assume that the protective activity of garlic oils may be due to the inhibition of lipid peroxidation by increasing GSH levels and reduction in the availability of O_2 for deleterious effects.

References

Adamu, I., Joseph, P.K. and Augusti, K.T. 1982: *Experientia*, 38: 899.

Aiyar, A.S. and De, A.K. 1978: *Strahlentherapie*, 154: 208.

Alprink, M.J. 1974: *Diabetes*, 23: 913.

Amenta, J.S. 1964: *J. Lipid Res.*, 5: 270.

Augusti, K.T. 1977: *Ind. J. Exp. Biol.*, 15: 489.

Ayene, S.I., Kale, R.K. and Srivastava, P.N. 1988: *Int. J. Radiat. Biol.*, 53: 629.

Ball, C.R. 1966: *Biohem. Pharmacol.*, 15: 809.

Baynen, A.C., Geelen, M.J.H. and Van den Bergh, S.G. 1980: *Trends Biochem. Sci.*, 5: 288.

Bindoli, A. 1988. Free Radiate. *Biol. Med.*, 5: 247.

Black, S. 1962: *Methos Enzymol.*, 5: 992.

Caldarera, M., Cozzani, F. and Moruzzi, M.S. 1966: *Experientia*, 22: 579.

Carison, L.A. and Bottiger, L.E. 1972: *Lancet.*, 1: 865.

Castro, J.A., De Ferreyra, G.C., De Castro, C.R., Sesame, H., De Fenos, O.M. and Gillette, J.R. 1974: *Bioichem Pharmacol.*, 23: 295.

Christophersen, B. D. 1968: *Biohem. J.*, 106: 515.

Christophersen, B.D. 1966: *Biohem. J.*, 100: 95.

Crawhall, J.C. and Watts, R.W.E. 1968: *Am. J. Med.*, 45: 736.

Cutier, R.G. 1991: *Am. J. Clin. Nutr.*, 53: 3735.

De, A.K. and Aiyar, A.S. 1978: *Strahlentherapie*, 154: 134.

Folch, J., Lees, M. and Sloane-Stanley, G.H. 1957: *J. Biol. Chem.*, 226: 497.

Gilbert, H.F. and Stewart, M.L. 1981: *J. Biol. Chem.*, 256: 1782.

Gupta, N.K. 1984: *Nat. Acad. Sci. Lett.*, 7: 285.

Gupta, N.K. 1990: *Medicina Nuclearis*, 2: 359.

Guyton, A.C. 1981: In Text Book of Medical Physiology (W.B. Saunders Co., Philadelphia, London, Toronto).

Halliwell, B., Gutteridge, J.M.C. and Cross, C.E. 1992: *J. Lab. Clin. Med.*, 199: 598.

Halliwell, B., Murcia, M.A., Chirico, S. and Aruoma, O. 1995: *Crit. Rev. Food Sci. Nutr.*, 35: 7.

Helzer, Z., Jozswiak, Z. and Leyko, W. 1980. *Experientia*, 36: 521.

Hodgson, E.K. and Fridovich, I. 1975: *Biochemistry*, 14: 5294.

Hepatic Disorders

Jain, M.K. and Apitz-Castrol, R. 1993: *Curr. Sci.*, 65: 148.

Kerognou, J.F., Braquet, M. and Rcoquet, G. 1981: *Radiat. Res.*, 88: 377.

Kolthoff, T.M., Stricks, W. and Kapoor, R.C. 1955: *J. Amer. Chem. So.*, 77: 4733.

Konings, A.W.T. and Drijver, E.B. 1979: *Radiat Res.*, 80: 479.

Kosower, N.S. and Kosower, E.M. 1976: In : Free radicals in Biology (ed. Pryor, W.) Academic Press. New York, Vol. III pp 55-84.

Natelson, S., In : Techniques of Clinical Chemistry (ed. Thomas, C.C., Public Spring Field, Illinois) 1971, 725.

Papas, A.M. 1996: *Lipids*, 31: S-77.

Petkau, A. and Chelak, W.S. 1976: *Biochem Biopys Acta.*, 443: 445.

Purohit, S.C., Bisby, R.H. and Cundali, R.B. 1980: *Int. J. Radiat. Biol.*, 38:147.

Rathi, A.B., Nath, N. and Chari, S.M. 1984: *Ind. J. Med. Res.*, 7: 508.

Releigh, J.A., Kremers, W. and Gaboury, B. 1977: *Int. J. Radiat. Biol.*, 31: 203.

Saghir, A.R., Mann, L.K., Bernhard, R.A. and Jacobson, J.V. 1964: *Proc. Am. Soc. Hort. Sci.*, 84: 386.

Silversmit, D.B. and Davis, A.K. 1950: *J. Lab. Clin. Med.*, 35: 155.

Skalka, M. 1958: *Nature,* 182: 1602.

Sodimu, O., Joseph, P.K. and Augusti, K.T. 1948: *Experientia*, 40: 78.

Temple, K.H. 1962: *Med. Ernahr.*, 3: 197.

Thomas, M.J. 1995: *Crit. Rev. Food Sci. Nutr.*, 35: 21.

Tretter, L., Ronai, E., Szabados, Gy., Hermann, R., Ando, A. and Horvath, I. 1990: *Int. J. Radiat. Biol.*, 57: 467.

Wills, E.D. and Wilkinson, A.E. 1970: *Int. J. Radiat. Biol.*, 17: 229.

Wooles, W.R. 1967: *Radiat. Res.*, 30: 788.

Yasuda, H., Izugami, N., Shamdar, P., Koba Yakawa, T. and Nakanishi, M. 1980. *Toxiol. Appl. Pharmacol.*, 52 : 407.

Yukawa, O. and Nakazawa, T. 1980: *Int. J. Radiat. Biol.*, 37: 621.

Yukawa, O., Miyahara, M., Shiraishi, N. and Nakazawa, T. 1985: *Int. J. Radiat. Biol.*, 48: 107.

Alterations in total lipids, triglycerides, phospholipids and free fatty acids in Mouse liver administred radiocalcium and their modification by Garlic oils

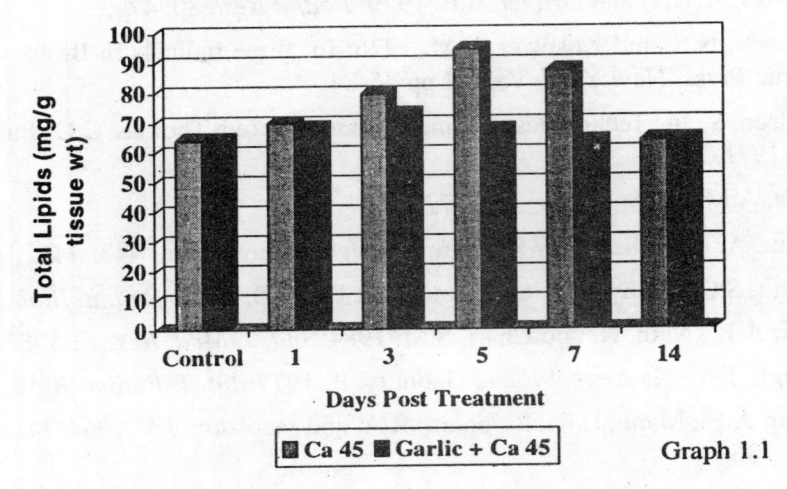

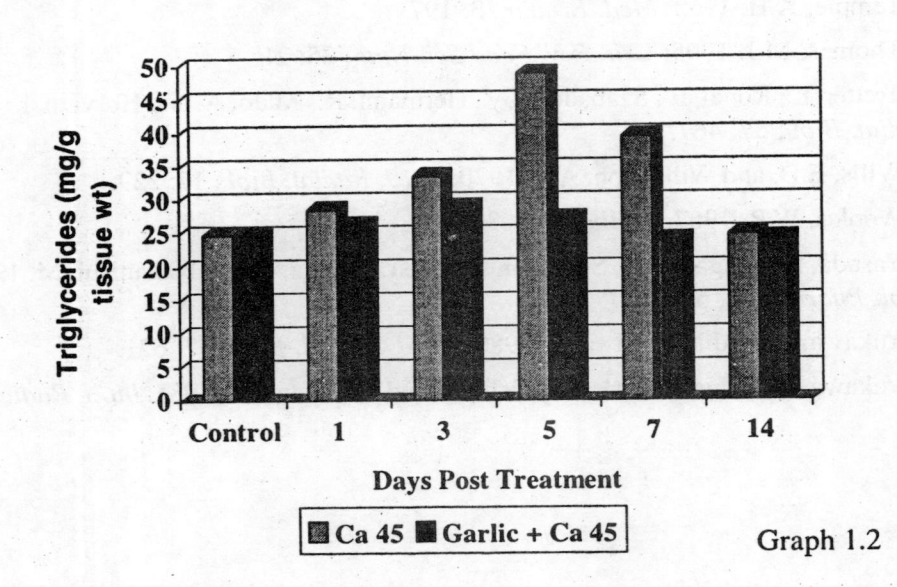

Graph 1.1

Graph 1.2

Hepatic Disorders

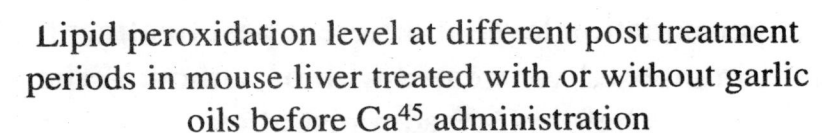

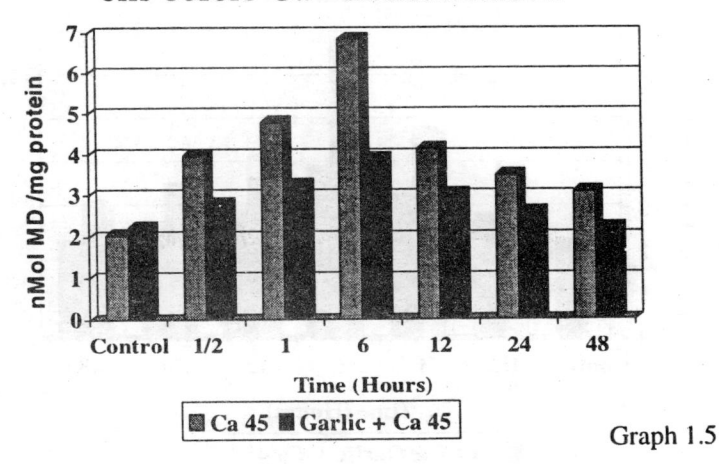

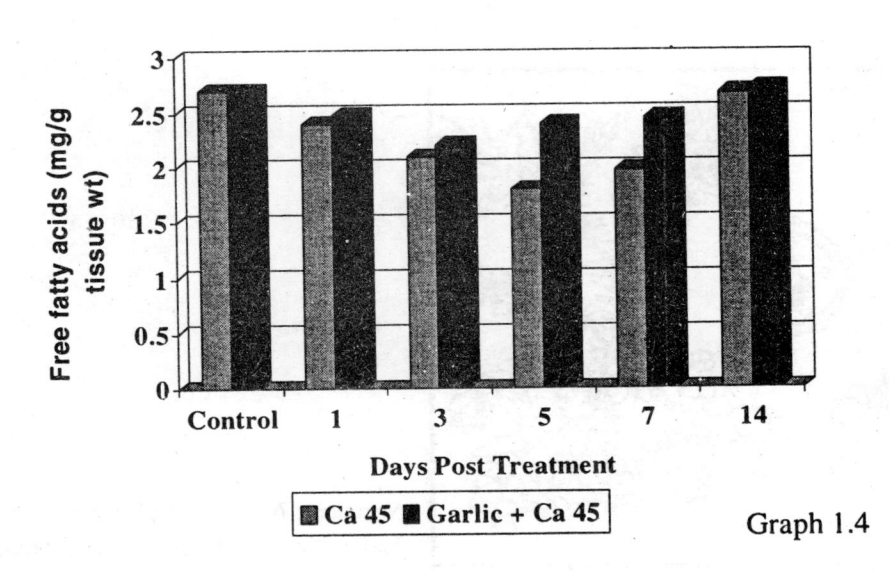

Lipid peroxidation level at different post treatment periods in mouse liver treated with or without garlic oils before Ca^{45} administration

Graph 1.5

Graph 1.4

Lipid peroxidation level at different post treatment periods in mouse liver treated with or without garlic oils before Ca^{45} administration

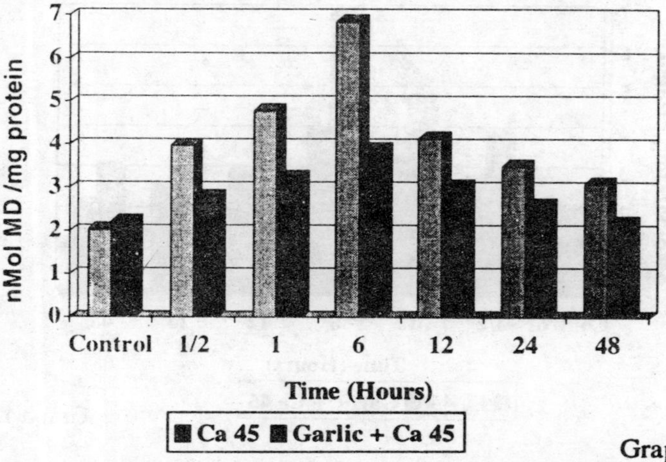
7
6
5
4
3
2
1
0
nMol MD /mg protein
Control
1/2
1
6
12
24
48
Time (Hours)
Ca 45
Garlic + Ca 45

Graph 1.5

Dr. Navneet K. Gupta
Dept. of Biology, College of Basic Sciences, H. P. Agricultural University, Palampur – 176062

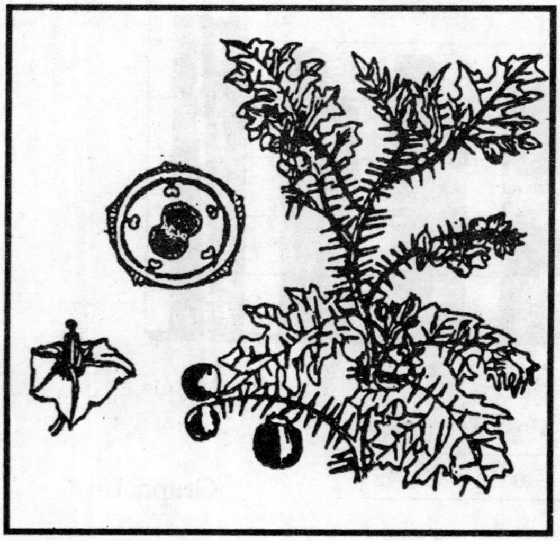

Sanskrit Name : Kantakari
Latin Name : Solanum xanthocarpum

Liver Dysfunction in Fetus : Hydrops Fetalis

Vd. Pradnya C. Nagnoor

Hydrops fetalis is the condition in which hepatic dysfunction causes symptoms. As far as Ayurvedic Literature is concerned, Yakruta is a moolasthana of Raktavaha srotasa and raktadhatu plays an important role in the development of fetus.

In Kasyapa Samhita, we get reference about development of organs originated from the raktadhatu.

S'onitatudhrutya tasya Jayate hridyadyakrit l

Yakruto Jayate Pleeha Pleehna : Phuphusamuchyate l l

Parsparanibandhani Sarvaniaetani Bhargava l

Kas'yapa Samhita

Sharirasthana

It means, heart, liver, spleen and lungs are formed from the raktadhatu.

Raktadhatu is a matruja dhatu and hence all above mentioned organs are matruja. In Modern Science, chronic anaemia leads to pathology of immune hydrops fetalis. The symptoms of Hydrops fetalis are pallor, generalised odema, hepatosplenomegaly etc. Garbha is a Rasaja and Pandu, Shotha are

Rasaprados'aja Vydhies, Raktadhatu is derived from Rasadhatu. Thus, we get correlation between Rasa, Rakta and Symptoms of Hydrops Fetalis.

Here we are discussing, the Immune Hydrops Fetalis which includes the pathology because

Hepatic Disorders

of liver dysfunction. In this, pathology starts from 'Rh' Incompatability which leads to excessive and prolonged haemolysis.

Pathology : According to Nicolini & Associates 1991

Stimulate marked erythroid Hyperplasia of Bone Marrow and large areas of extra medullary haem Atopoiesis i.e. liver and spleen

Excessive and Prolonged Haemolysis
⇩
Profound Anaemia
⇩
Tissue Hypoxia
⇩
Decreased Colloid on Cotic pressure
⇩
Hypoprotinemia

⇩ Causes

Hepatic Dysfunction
⇩
Portal and umbilical venous hypertension from hepatic parenchymal disruption by extramedullary haematopoieses.

Symptoms :

- Considerable generalised subcutaneous odema and effusion into the serous cavities.
- Hepatosplenomegaly.
- Ascites
- Cardiac enlargement
- Fetus shows 'Buddha' Position in straight X-Ray Abdomen. It is because of odematous scalp.
- Placenta = Marketdly edematous, enlarged
  Boggy
  Edematous villi
  Large, prominent cotyledons
- Fetuses with hydrops may die in utero from profound anaemia and

Hepatic Disorders

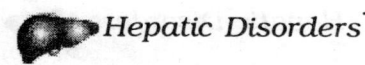

circulatory failure.

❏ The baby is either stillborn or macerated and even if born alive dies soon after.

Diagnosis :

• Diagnosis is easily made with the help of ultrasonography as severe edema is easily identified by USG.

• Previous obstestric History also helps to diagnose Hydrops Fetalis.

e.g. bad Obstetric History which includes known case of Rh Incompatability.

• Intrauterine Death

• Stillbirth

• Neonatal Death because of severe jaundice.

Histological Examination of liver :

◆ Fatty degenerative parenchymal changes.

◆ Deposition of hemosiderin.

◆ Engorgement of hepatic canaliculi with bile.

Investigations :

To study this pathology Nicolaidas and colleagues performed Percutaneous Umbilical Artery Blood Sampling in 17 severely 'D' isoimmunised fetuses at 18 to 25 wks of gestation (In 1985)

1. All fetuses with hydrops had Hb values of less than 3.8 g/dl.
2. Plasma Protein concentration less than 2 standard deviations from the mean for normal fetuses of ascitic fluid.
3. Fetoscopy = Substantive protein concentrations in ascitic fluid.

These investigations concluded that the degree and duration of anaemia influence the severity of ascites and this is made worse by hypoprotenemia.

The effect of lesser form of fetal haemolysis is Icterus Gravis Neonatorum. The baby is born alive without evidences of jaundice but soon develops it within 24 hrs. of birth.

While the fetus is in utero, there is destruction of fetal red cells with liberation of unconjugated bilirubin which is mostly excreted through the placenta into the maternal system. A portion of the bilirubin enters the amniotic fluid perhaps from the fetal lung or through the skin or across the surface of the placenta or cord. This is the reason why the baby is not born with jaundice.

But as soon as the umbilical cord is clamped with continuing harmolysis,

Hepatic Disorders

the bilirubin concentration is incresed. Sooner or later the baby becomes jaundiced. The liver, particularly of a premature baby fails to conjugate the excessive amount of bilirubin to make it soluble and non-toxic.

If the bilirubin rises to the critical level of 20 mg / 100 ml, the bilirubin crosses the blood-brain barrier to damage the basal nuclei of the brain permanently producing the clinical manifestation of kernicterus.

In Hydrops fetalis, premature labour is common. In premature babies, jaundice becomes on early and is often very deep because the liver is unable to remove bile constitutents from the blood sufficiently readily, as there is low albumin levels and consequent reduction in bilirubin binding capacity. In Immune Hydrops Fetalis, this condition is more severe as the rate of haemolysis is more severe as the rate of haemolysis is more than other premature babies.

According to Protocol, such cases of hydrops fetalis are advised to be terminated. But it is necessary to avoid successive hydrops pregnancies. For that, we get prophylactic management for immune hydrops fetalis such as

1. To avoid fetomaternal bleed during delivery, caeserian section etc. in Rh-'ve' mother and Rh+'ve' father, so that chances of being isoimmunised get reduced.

2. After delivery and abortion, Injectable Anti-'D' to the mother having Rh-'ve' group and baby having Rh+'ve' group.

From Ayurvedic Point of View, a thought behind hydrops fetalis is, there may be imbalance between Teja and Aapa Mahabhoota which influence the pathology. This thought may be helpful in the treatment of hydrops fetalis. But this needs a lot of research.

It also necessary to get ayurvedic paribhasa and samprapti for antibodies which causes haemolysis. Is it possible to reduce the rate of haemolysis by herbal drug ? either by Rasaprasadaka or Raktaprasadaka or Mahabhautic chikitsa and hence it is a research work for us.

Vd. Pradnya C. Nagnoor, M. D. IIIrd year (Gyn-Obst)
Tilak Ayurved Mahavidyalaya

Horoscope and Liver Disorders

Dr. Shrikant Bhide

As per medical astrology, organ liver and its condition can be judged by the 5 th house of the Basic Horoscope or Janmalagna kundali

1. 5th house also indicates stomach area, epigastric, hypochondriac part of the body.

2. Planet mars, sun and jupiter tells about the condition of the liver and its all functions. As these planets indicate condition of pitta dosha i.e. pachakpitta in the body.

3. Condition of the sign Leo and its lord Sun also tells about condition of liver and bile / pachak pitta.

4. In diseased condition, the lord of the 6 th house and 1st house they come in relation of 5 th house.

5. Regarding prognosis, Mahadasha / period of the planets in relation with 5 th or 11th house and sign lord, that used the clue about good or the bad prognosis of the disease.

6. The affected planets also give idea about the complications e.g. Hepatic coma, hepatitis etc.

7. So before onset of the disease, we can use medical astrology as a preventive measure, as we can trace the weaker liver function before onset of the liver disorder.

Dr. Shrikant N. Bhide
6/63 Tulashibagwale Colony, Hemavati Apartments, 1 st Floor, Sahakar Nagar- 2,
Pune-411009, Tel- 422-5536

HEPATIC COMA – AYURVEDIYA MANAGEMENT

Vd. M. D. Sane.

Hepatic Coma or precoma is a clinical syndrome characterized by neuropsychiatric complications followed by failure of Liver cells. Liver is an organ of Raktavah. Srotas and is made up in foetal Life from important 'Dhatu' Rakta. This condition occurs when the products of intestinal absorption (raised Ammonia) reach the brain, either because they are not metabolized by Rakta dhatu agni or because of portal systemic as in chronic cell failure. Rasadhatu or Ahar – Ras is the substance that goes to liver and Rakta is produced.

Viral – Toxic or drug induced hepato cellular necrosis results into Hepatic Coma. Chronic Hepatic encephalopathy occurs due to portal caval shunts either intra hepatic (cirrhosis) or prehepatic (cirrhosis, portal vein thrombosis and therapeutic).

In cirrhosis of Liver hepatic coma may be precipitated by severe upper gastrointestinal hemorrhage as in Urdhwaga – Rakta – Pitta, fluid and electrolyte imbalances, following excessive diuretic therapy – (especially Thiazides) and rapid abdominal paracentesis, systemic infection, renal failure, high protein diet, alcoholic bouts and surgery, intra abdominal disease (acute pancreatitis and constipation. One more important precipitating factor is the use of drugs that are primarily metabolized in liver e. g. Morphine, pethidine, barbiturates and paraldehyde.

Though the mechanism of production of hepatic coma is not clearly understood, Hepatocellular failure and portal systemic shunts contribute to the genesis of hepatic encephalopathy by allowing nitrogenous products of bacterial fermentation in colon, take ammonia to reach brain, which is sensitive to their toxic actions. The rate of branched chain aminoacids to aromatic aminoacids act as weak neurotransmitters and may displace normal neurotransmitters in brain. Such as adrenaline and dopamine and thus produce hepatic coma.

Quantitative increase in blood results in 'Sammoh' as clinical feature according to Ayurvedic

Hepatic Disorders

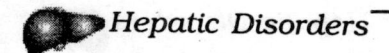

texts. This leads to irritability, alterations in personality, inability to do simple arithmetic either addition or subtraction, confusion and insomnia.

Speech is slurred and handwriting becomes difficult and illegible. A peculiar disagreeable odour is of particular diagnostic value. "Nishwas – Vaigandhya" is specifically described sign in ayurvedic texts is much more similar to this sign.

This followed by lethargy, flapping tremous, (inability to maintain posture) stupor and finally loss of consciousness, uremia and co_2 necrosis can be ruled out in some patients. Decerebrate and Decorticate rigidity may also develop in some terminal stages of Hepatic Coma.

Electro Encephalogram may show characteristic symmetrical high voltage slow waves in hepatic Coma.

Other features of this disease include
1) Jaundice
2) Gynaecomastia
3) Hepatomegaly
4) Spleenomegaly
5) Ascites

Principles of the treatment
a) Maintain Electrolyte balance.
b) High protein Diet be avoided
c) Constipation to be treated.
d) Upper Gastrointestinal Bleeding be stopped.
e) Accurate antibiotics
f) Neomycin or stapromycin be given
g) Lactulose
h) Fresh blood transfusions.

Ayurved may be of importance in treatment of Hepatic or prehepatic Coma.

1) Nasya - of Haridra & Daru haridra quath may help in reducing Ammonia saturation in Encephalopathy.

2) Basti - (Type of Enema) of Dashmoot quath and saindhava in pinchful quantity may be useful to reduce toxicity in guts.

Hepatic Disorders

3) Sugarcane Juice - and Laaja mand. May maintain electrolytic balance.

4) वासा गुडूचि त्रिफला कडी भूनिंब निंबजा

क्वाथः क्षौद्र युतोः

Vasa may help gastrointestinal bleeding stoppage. Guduchi will act as an antibiotic in guts.

Triphala and Kutki act for correct management of Constipation.

Bhunimb and Nimb helps in regeneration of liver cells.

Honey acts as alternative treatment to Lactulose.

Clinical trials and Correct research method may be useful to determine the effects of this treatment.

During the treatment Nonveg diet should be avoided.

Dr. M. D. Sane
12, Kohinoor Complex, 5th Floor, V. N. Purao Marg, Chembur Naka, Mumbai – 400 071
Tel : 5585306 (O), 5561070 (R)

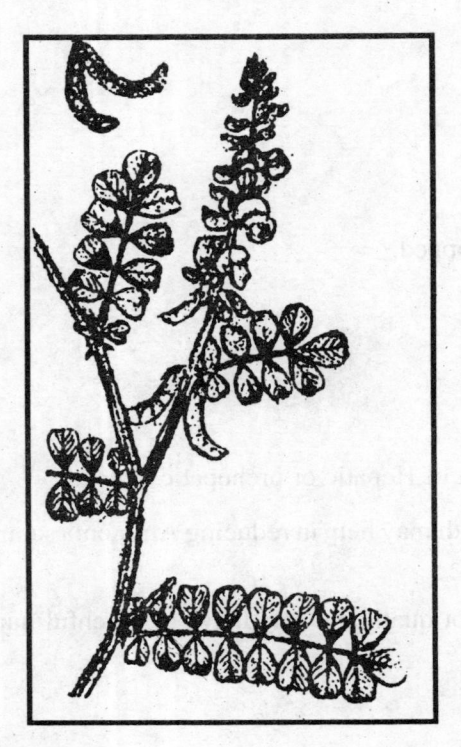

Sanskrit Name : Sharapunkha
Latin Name : Tephrosia purpurea

Hepatic Disorders

Roll Of Yakrita In Apasmara Chikitsa

Vd. Vivek Sudhakar Haldavnekar

Introduction

Man has always tried to seek different solutions for his problems. Let it be health problems or other. Apasmar is one of those problem, which has made Vaidyas / Doctors always alert to seek some solutions. Moreover this is the disease, which one has to see in his practice in two stages viz. Status & Non status, Here we have tried to solve this problem using PanchaBhoutik Chikitsa as its base.

Yakrit (Liver)

This is a prime organ based on the right side of the body. It is the main sthan (base) for 'Pachaka Pitta'. The Grahani sthit Agni or Kayagni is also represented by this 'Pachak Pitta', Mainly Aahar rasa or Rasa Dhatu get treated with this 'Pitta' to form 'Rakta Dhatu'. Some Pachak Pitta while running through all over body is called accordingly sadhak, Ranjak, Bhrajak & Aalochak Pitta as per its different functions.

Apasmar

According to Ayurvedic texts Apsmar is seen due to disturbances in working of 'Udana Vayu'. Functions described of 'Udana Vayu' are बलवर्णस्मृतीक्रिय: वा.

Udana gets covered by vitiated 'Kapha' & 'Pitta'. This vitiation of kapha & Pitta is mainly due to lack of working of liver.

" अपसार निदान - चिंताशोकादिभिर्दोषा: कृद्धा हृत्स्त्रोतांसि रिथता:

कृत्वा स्मृतेरपध्वंसमपरमारं प्रकुर्वते । " यो.र.

Hepatic Disorders

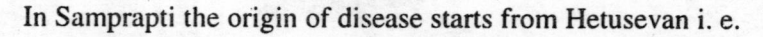

In Samprapti the origin of disease starts from Hetusevan i. e.

चिंताशोकादिभि: मानस भाव:

But these cases are mostly seen in children where these causes are rarely present or mostly absent. In most of these cases. We have treated, the Nidan or Hetu of disease (Atiology) is mainly history of 'Kamala' present in victims or in their mothers during pregnancy. In 'Kamala' the 'Rakta Dhatu' mainly get vitiated due to increased 'Teja mahabhut' i.e. 'Pitta'.

प्रलापभूच्छ्रंभ्रमपित्तदाहा: पित्तस्य कर्मणी वदन्ति तज्ज्ञा : । यो.र.

So here the disease originates from 'Sharir', then leads to 'Manas Vyadhi'. Because the already vitiated 'Rasa & Rakta Dhatu nourish all the body & also mind.

While treating these cases, first 'Pachan Vyapar' must be corrected. So liver is the main functioning part to take carefully. The main drug used to correct liver metabolism is 'Phala Trikadi Guggul'.

Phala trikadi guggul - Main contents are Triphala, Kutki, Kirattikta, Vasa, Nimb, Guduchi. Here Kutki does Bhedan karma & distroys 'Dosha vibandha' with the help of triphala by virechan. Triphala & Guduchi both do 'Rasayan' karma. All these combinations help to correct the flow of Pitta in natural form & regains 'Samyavastha of Tridosha'.

Here it won't be improper to mention that no text mentioned Antiepileptic drugs were used in this study, till No. of patients were cured with this treatment.

Vd. Vivek Sudhakar Haldavnekar
38, L. I. C. Colony, Kawala Naka, Tararani Chowk, Kolhapur.
Clinic – 667464, Resi. – 654597, E-mail -vivh@pn3.vsnl.net.in

Hepatic Disorders

Herbal Applications In The Treatment Of Hepatic Aspects In Human Life

G. S. Chandras.
Mrs. Sunetra Gokhale.

1. It is most appropriate that this year's Seminar on Ayurved has "the Liver" as its leading theme.

2. In the 1920s, 1930s and 1940s, diseases like Malaria, Cholera, Tuberculosis etc. were very rampant. They took a heavy toll in our society. During the 1980s and 1990s, it seems that Diabetes, Blood Pressure, Heart Attacks and Cancer were overriding us on a significant scale. During 1990s in particular, the "AIDS" has made a prominent appearance on our scene.

3. But it appears now that in the next two decades, we may suffer colossal causalities on account of problems of "Liver". Liver is believed to produce blood out of the foods and other intakes. Liver is supposed to be a sealed unit, the working of which seems difficult to understand.

Liver is the largest and the most important gland in our body. It is well known to be useful to us on the following counts :

a) Production of blood
b) Production of vital body elements
c) Proper digestion of foods etc.
d) Secretion of bile and storage of glycogen
e) Mobilization of proteins and fats etc.

Mal-functioning of Liver can cause Jaundice, Cirrhosis and also inefficiency in our body – functioning in a number of ways.

4. The importance of Liver seems to have been recognized thousands of years ago.

Hepatic Disorders

For example – the saint "Chyavan" is said to have regained his Youth mainly on the strength of his Liver :-

"यकृन: हृदय समीपे वर्तमान: कालमांस विशेष तस्मात यकृत ' ऋग्वेद

Liver is said to have worked many other wonders in innumerable cases mentioned in old Sanskrit Literature.

5. In present era, a total revolution in our food habits has arrived in striking contrast to ideal diet. Burgers, Pizzas, Wada-Pav, Bread, Cakes, Pastries, Farsans, Chocolates, Sandwiches, heavy sweets, Ice Creams, Fried preparations etc. are becoming more and more popular, in the young generation. Drinking Alcohol has become a prestigious style. Coca-Cola, Pepsi, Thumps-up, Limca, Sprite, Mangola etc. are taking a grip over the youth.

Poultry Farms and Goat Farms are sprawling all over. Difficult to digest and Spicy food are becoming increasingly popular. The days of Rice, Dal, Vegetables and Curds are fading in the background. The importance of roughage is being grossly ignored.

As if this is not enough, other factors e.g. A) The Rising Level of Mental Stress, B) Pollution in the Air, Foods and Water etc. will be making the job of the Liver still more difficult. The outcome seems to be obvious. The health level in the society is bound to degenerate and "Health is Wealth" will remain only a slogan in the Air.

6. On the other hand the Therapeutic Forces, Structures and Organizations seem to be lagging far behind the aggression by the Major Ailments of the present times. Medical colleges and Research Institutes admit that they are still not aware of the causes of Cancer, which has already killed innumerable Cancer Patients. The same is the cause about AIDS also. We are likewise forced to admit that we have no guaranteed cure on CANCER OR AIDS.

7. At this stage we are reminded of the Great French Thinker **VOLTAIRE** who said that :-

"DOCTORS PRESCRIBE DRUGS OF WHICH THEY KNOW LITILE,

INTO BODIES OF WHICH THEY KNOW NOTHING"

But all the same, we need doctors because we cannot manage ourselves when ill. Our illness is mostly caused due to our mistakes, bad habits, our outlooks and our attitudes. Alternative therapies with exaggerated and fluctuating claims are continuously evolving, which makes a judicious choice between Therapies and Doctors very tricky. Eventually, we are playing with our own life and money. Any ill treatment or injustice to the Liver seems to send out signals to our body and mind. We should not therefore ignore such signals from the Liver, though it appears generally, that the symptoms of ill treatment or injustice to Liver are detected rather late with consequent Complications. Sufferance and expenses.

Hepatic Disorders

8. But the case of Liver ailments seems to be much more serious as compared to that of Cancer and AIDS. Hepatitis – B is said to be hundred times more infectious than AIDS. Hepatitis – B is said to kill more people in a day than AIDS kills in a year. There is nothing in view to cure Hepatitis – B. We are therefore strongly advised to take vaccines to protect ourselves from an attack of hepatitis – B. So "PREVENTION IS BETTER THAN CURE"

9. If we are agreeable to learning from the experiences of the past, on the aspect of Liver, we like to bring to your notice a few of the references we could easily find out of the old Sanskrit Literature. Perhaps these references have behind them the wisdom of time – tested treatments. They are old, bug let us look at them with an open mind and accept them or not on the basis of our own studies, tests, experiments etc. in the interest of our future.

10. Herbs mentioned to be useful in treatment of Liver.

Zingiber Officinale	Piper Nigrum
Trachyspermum sp.	Piper longum
Ferula foetida	Euryale ferox
Terminalia arjuna	Woodfordia fruticosa
Achyaranthes aspera	Musa paradisiaca
Sesamum indicum	Eleusine caracana
Datura metel	Curcuma longa
Bambusa arundinacea	Ficus bengalensis
Curcuma zedoaria	Asparagus racemosus
Terminalia chebula	Azadirachta indica
Ocimum sanctum	Artocarpus heterophyllus
Jasmimum grandiflorum	Berberis aristata
Rubia cordifolia	Raulfia serpentina
Mimusops elengi	Zizyphus mauritiana

11. Ayurvedic preparations for treatments in Liver disorders :-

चित्रकादि चूर्ण	वडनावल चूर्ण	कुमारी आसव
यवानी खाण्डव चूर्ण	अजमोदादि चूर्ण	गोमुत्र क्षार
हिंग्वादी चूर्ण	स्वादिष्ट विरेचण चूर्ण	नवायस चूर्ण
शुष्ठ्यादी चूर्ण	अमृतारिष्ट	लघुमालिनी वसंत
तुम्बुर्वादी चूर्ण	रोहितकारिष्ट	आरोग्यवर्धिनी

Hepatic Disorders

12. Other Remedies

a) Eating of preparations of Liver For maintenance of Liver, preparations of Liver of other animals are eaten. It has been stated that :- अति

b) Sprouted Grains etc :- Sprouts of wheat, cereals, rise etc have been known to be beneficial for increasing efficiency of Liver.

c) Butter Milk :- ButterMilk has been known to be helpful in improving the digestive system.

It is a well-known phrase :

तर्कं शक्रस्य दुर्लभम्

Which means that ButterMilk cannot be enjoyed by the Gods because ButterMilk is produced out of spoiled milk and nothing gets spoiled in the Heavens.

13. Plantations in Shivanand Enclave, Pune :

We have before us plans for plantations of important Medicinal Plants. We have adequate lands on the outskirts of Pune for this purpose. We welcome participation in this programme.

14. Web-site :

In the present age of Information Technology, today's Seminar may consider establishment of a Web-site specially for the patients and Doctors concerned with the problems of Liver, if it has not been already established in the World. This will facilitate exchange of notes and experiences on the subjects of Liver – Management.

G. S. Chandras. (Botany graduate 1947, Indian Forest Service till 1977, Head of the forestry Economics Division at Gokhale Institute of Politics and economics, Pune. Presently engaged in establishing gardens of medicinal plants near Pune.)
Mrs. Sunetra Gokhale. (B. A. LL. B. from Pune. Custodian of the Gardens in Shivanand Enclave near Pune.)

Hepatic Disorders

The Urgent For Hepatitis B Vaccination

Dr. S. Bhardwaj & Dr. S.V. Kapre

Abstract

Hepatitis B is an acute systemic infection with major pathology in the liver and accounts for 2 billion infected individuals globally and 350 million chronic carriers. The mortality is about 1-2 million deaths per year. In 5-15% cases HBV infection fails to resolve leading persistent carriers, which lead to Chronic Active Hepatitis and Primary Liver Cancer. Due to the lack of specific treatment, Prevention is the major aim in management. Recombinant Hepatitis B vaccine is available in India and is being used for immunization. The vaccine has also been introduced in the Universal Immunization Schedule as a pilot project in Delhi State. In order to reduce the current prevalence of carriers the Vaccine need to be used on a larger scale specially in the high risk groups like male homosexuals, neonates and infants, adolescents with multiple sexual partners, I V drug abusers, Health Care personnel, Prisoners and International Travelers. The Hepatitis B Vaccine is given in a dose of 1 ml. I/M containing 20 micro-grams of HbsAg per dose. The Vaccine is administered in three doses at 0.1 and 6 months. An effective antibody response is attained after 3 doses in about 95% of Vaccines. Booster dose may be given after 3-5 years. HBIG (immunoglobulin) can be combined with the Vaccine and is ideal for prophylaxis of persons accidentally exposed to blood known to contain Hepatitis B Virus and for prevention of carrier state in Newborn babies of carrier mothers. The dose of HBIG is 0.05-0.07 ml/kg of body weight 2 doses given 30 days apart. Additionally it is absolutely essential to incorporate Hepatitis B Vaccine for mass use in the National Immunization Programme as has been effectively done by more than 75 countries worldwide.

Dr. S. Bhardwaj & Dr. S.V. Kapre
Serum Institute Of India Ltd, Pune

Vasadi Kashayam - My Drug of Choice in Kamala (Hepatitis)

Dr. Atulchandra Thombre

It was rather my previlage & pleasure, that I got an opportunity to treat & help thomands of patients with Ayurveda. Out of them hundred of patients were suffering from either malfunctioning or a diseased liver.

MAlfunctioning of liver can cause improper digestion i.e. Ajeerna, which in turn leads to innumerable diseases, by producing Amma i.e. undigested Rasadhatu and that is the reason why it is of immense importance to treat the malfunctioning of the liver at the earliest.

According to my 16 years of practise opinion the unique formulation for Hepatitis is 'Vasadi kashayan' (Ref. Asthanga Hridayam)

Following are the ingredients of Vasadi Kashayam

1. Vasa 2. Guduchi 3. Triphala 4. Katuka 5. Bhunimba 6. Nimba

Indication by experience

Apart from the excellent efficacy of Vasadi Kashayam stated in Phalashriti of the kashayam. I have successfully used this prolific formulation in following Hepatic Disorders-

1. Malfunctioning of liver causing anorexia & indigestion.

2. All types of Udara roga, especially in yakrut dalyodar & pleehodara.

3. Udar purvarupavastha.

4. Yakrut sankoch i.e. liver cirhosis etc.

This combination of kashayam is extremely effective in both the subtypes of kamala as it promotes the proper secretion of pitta into the small intensive is responsible for expelling out

Hepatic Disorders

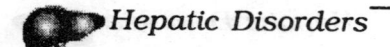

the disease causing vitiated pitta dosha by its virechaka or purgative action.

Vasadi kashayam curtail and cure almost all the signs and symptoms in kamala and malfunctioning of liver as well. Another charismatic characterstic of vasadi kashayam is it can be used either Shaman or Shodhana.

By mixing c Honey it can be given as shaman chikitsa & for the shodhan chikitsa we have to take all three ingredients triphala separately and double the part of Katuka.

To over come the 'Bitter taste' one can add some binding agent like gum acacia and prepaare its tablets or one may fill the powder of kashayam ingredients in capsules.

To increase the potency of the drug and to reduce its dose one can triturate the powder of kashayam with its own decoction one can ad guggulu in it.

Being as herbal preparation it is absolutely safe it is almost harmless and non-hazardous to the patterns

---

Vd. Atulchandra S. Thombare
96, D-2/B-3, Dixit Baug App., Sagamnerkar Hospital Lane, Navi Peth, Pune – 411 030
Tel : 4331492 (O), 4354884 (R)

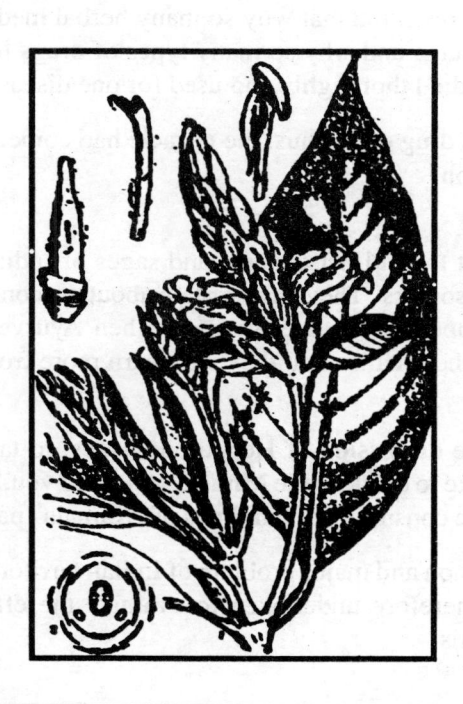

Sanskrit Name : Vasa
Latin Name : Adhatoda vasica

Clinical Assessment Of Effect Of Kamalant In "Kamala"

Dr. Manohar J. Karachiwala.

Introduction

I am practicing as a general practitioner in Ahmednagar since 1986. I had passed my B.Sc. from Pune University in Zoology securing 78% marks [First class with Distinction] in 1979 & B.A.M.S. from Nagpur University in 1984 and started my general practice from 1986.

While studying Ayurved, I have a point in my mind that why so many herbal medicines combination are made to make a single medicine and why so many types of drugs for one disease? Why not a single drug should be studied thoroughly and used for one disease.

Thus, this was my first step towards single drug use. Thus, the miracle had come up my thinking, I started my research in this direction.

Aims And Objectives

The treaties of Ayurved clearly tell us that the old, wise saints and sages of India were aware of the problem of Liver Diseases and Disorders. They have written about the condition, it's etiological factors and the treatment proper. Gone are the days when Ayurved was looked down by the learned and wise. Now they realise that they will learn more from this ancient science of health and healing.

Dear friends, here we are gathered for the discussion of Hepatic damages; to take the chance of this Golden opportunity, I would like to disclose the Miracle of herb to you, which I obtained from my 14 years special Ayurvedic consulting of hundreds of "Kamala" patients.

"KAMALA" is one of the epidemic, common and major problem of Indian territory such as Ahmednagar District. This study was therefore undertaken to evaluate the effect of "KAMALANT" in "KAMALA" i.e. Hepatitis

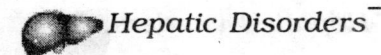

Hepatic Disorders
Material
Generally, Kamalant is used in liquid form. And, I used 1gm. Of Herbal medicine diluted in 10 ml. simple water as a standard dose.

Doses :   200 ml. = For Adults

100 ml. = For Children 5 to 13 years.

50 ml. = For Children below 5 years.

25 ml. = For Infants

Administration : Single dose daily, preferably, early in the morning to take the advantage of empty stomach for maximum absorption of the medicine.

Anupan : Sugar is added as per requirement of taste.

No. of Kamala Patients / subjects – 25

Serum Bilirubin profile and Urine Bile salt + pigment was done before and after Kamalant treatment.

Methodology
I have classified the "Kamala" patients into two groups according to pathological profile of serum Bilirubin.

1. Direct Serum Bilirubin level : Which generally raised due to Intra-hepatic factors i.e. Viral or infective or obstructive

2. Indirect Serum Bilirubin level : Which generally raised due to Extra-hepatic factors i.e. Haemolitic

Effect Of Kamalant Treatment On Serum Bilirubin Profile
Nineteen (19) patients shows excellent response to the drug given to them only within 4 days / doses.

On the other extent, Six (6) patients shows moderate response to the drug given to them even after 7 days / doses.

Results And Discussions
·· Kamalant is effective upto 76%.

·· Moderately for 24%

·· Kamalant is most effective in Intra-hepatic cases rather than Extra-hepatic cases.

·· Actually it is my thinking that generally Kamala is due to thickening of BILE i.e. Pitta its viscosity comes down due to Viral infection thus there is no free flow of bile to the

Duodenum and some tomes due to more thickening it gets blocked up, thus it appears to be obstructive Jaundice, but in USG no obstruction is seen. Thus the colour of the stool changes to white. (Tilkalk).

Kamalant when taken taken orally nil by mouth it directly goes through the common bile duct to the thickened bile and it liquefies bile, thus the bile is again free flown into the Duodenum and thus result.

Dr. Manohar J. Karachiwala.
B.Sc., B.A.M.S. –Dept. of Preventive & Clinical Medicine Dr. Chavan Hospital & Research Centre., Ahmednagar.

Hepatic Disorders

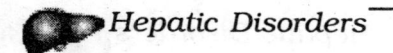

Health Is A State Which We Create

Swami Joythirmayanand

Purpose of this paper is to share my experience of the last 20 years in the field of helping people to improve their life quality by taking care of their organs such as liver.

In my view the liver is not just a physical organ, but I like to think of it as a whole with a physical level, also a mental, an intellectual and even a spiritual level. This is the thought I would like to share with you this year.

Liver
Liver is the mother earth

How the mother earth transforms the seed into a beautiful plant, flowers and fruits, in the same way the liver has the ability to transform the food into useful vital energy. I see the liver as whole in various levels : physical, mental, intellectual and also spiritual.

Physical level

The liver transform food into body cells of basic 5 elements. Thus they flow all through the body and nourish each and every tissue, as well as other organs. Similarly the liver digests toxic food, which keep it by protecting other cells and organs from the effect of such harmful elements. Thus we can imagine, from the physiological viewpoint, the liver as the protecting and nourishing constituent of our body.

Mental level

The mental viewpoint address our interest to consider how liver, which remain the first filter of our body, can manage with happiness, stress, power and fatigues. Emotion derived from such a living condition influence the liver, and the liver play an important role in transforming such emotion into physiological improvement when positive emotion are lived, or malfunction when negative emotion is the condition of the subject.

Hepatic Disorders

Intellectual level

The next step regards the way how the liver may transfer emotion into physiological activity, or how it may manage emotion by receiving good or bad food. This depends on the intellectual level which I like to consider in this paper. The ability of the liver to digest anger or jealousy without leading to major pathological body condition is an ability which is proper of the single individual. Similarly the ability of determination or courage of a subject is coming from the intellectual properties of the subject, and the liver, using its own intellect, becomes the organs which gives the energy which is necessary to maintain such a courage or power.

Spiritual level

Finally the ability of our liver to put in harmony the different incoming signals which it receive is its spiritual level. Naturally the flow of the body is well designed in harmonious way, because it is flowing only in the presence. It is the health state.

Everything goes within a energy level and this energy is controlled by an intelligence. Each and every individual has his own perfect intelligence, which is part of the cosmic existence. We could feel this infinite cosmic experience whenever we go beyond the individual body, where there is no disease nor suffering, no good nor bad, no stress nor fatigue. This is the cosmic intelligence. The body itself, each and every part of it and its memory is part of this cosmic intelligence when the human being is living this status he is healthy and well being. But it is not always so. Sometimes disease comes and I would express my thought of the path toward disease.

Life stile is the disease

Life stile is the disease : because of the illusion, an individual may get off from his present, and try to live in his past or future. This is done by himself with the purpose of improving his life, indeed this is the way to reduce harmony in himself because the individual identify his imagination of reality as his reality ... he is out of presence. This is the primary causes of disease as lack of harmony with the nature and present moment.

The cause for the disease

This loss of harmony reflect on the intellect of the individual. As the intellect is affected by existential uncertainty, its constituent, such as ego, may become mad inducing conflict which decrease the ability of the body, and thus also the liver, to manage with incoming components such as food and emotion. In this condition, a bad food might more easily determine a toxic effect in the body able to lead to a pathological condition, similarly, a normal behavior of another person can be misunderstood by the individual. Thus physical and mental levels may be damaged by the spiritual and intellectual levels. In this sense I consider the progress toward disease and pathological condition of liver or whichever organ of the body.

Hepatic Disorders

The Treatment

I like to focus an aspect of the intellect which I manage in treatments : it is the personality of the individual. In this sense I consider disease strongly dependent on the personality of the individual. Each personality has its own disease. Each and every organ try to bear the error of the intellectual and spiritual levels, according to their bearing capacity. On behalf of protecting the superior organ, the intelligence of the liver, bear the emotional and intellectual disharmony leading to a pathological condition and the corresponding life style.

Thus pathological condition may occur and treatment becomes necessary. My view is again the uncommon sight which require the whole change of the person, not the resolution of a symptom, together with proper diet and drugs according to the physicians I work with.

For the diet, in case of liver problems, my suggestion is to take hot (acid) and cold (alkaline) energy food in different meals; in particular I suggest hot food at lunch and cold food at dinner.

Correcting habitual life style is the treatment

The philosophy of the treatment is the individual rebuilding of an harmonious life style. I ask my patients to change his life style routine in positive manner. Good routine help to balance ones nature, and consequentially the personality will elevate to Satvic state.

The method which I use is in the following. I utilize *activity, nourishment and rest* through the practices of Yoga, Ayurveda and a method I elaborated, which I called "NYM" or "Nome-Yantra-Mantra".

The aim of my practice is to teach self-correcting methods to everybody. The principles of the methods are the same for healthy and sick persons. By practicing, they strength themselves and become able to perceive the environment in a more positive way. The techniques are totally harmless, and prepare the person to keep alert and happy with satisfactory results. The self correcting method is at the level of : soul, intellect, emotion, energy and physical body. Instruments are : purification, relaxation, fortification, maintaining a pure identity. The main aim is : peace, health and happiness.

Yoga
Panchanga Yoga

1. *Asana* and *Pranayama* for the strength and health of the body.
2. *Banda* and *Mudra* for the study and balance of the energy.
3. *Mantra* and *Japa* for the perception of unity and peaceful emotion.
4. *Darshana* and *Satsang* for the clarity of intellect.
5. *Dharana* and *Dhiyana* for the well beings of the soul.

Ayurvedic techniques

- **Abyanga**

Daily, fortnight and monthly

- **Panchakarma treatment**

Twice in a year

- **Specific diet according to constitution (Prakruti)**

Prepare fresh and clean food;

Eat small but balanced quantity of food in scheduled time;

Never overeat and avoid pecking;

Eat when there is ideal hunger, with empty stomach and having a good desire to eat. While eating keep in tranquillity and happy;

After eating feel the maximum of satisfaction.

- **Remedies for detoxification, Relaxation and Rajuvenation**

I personally specialized and successfully experimented three ayurvedic preparations to these aims:

> Niragada decoction to detoxify (main ingredients : Tripala, Trikatu ....),
> Shanti infusion to relax (main ingredients : Brahmmi, Shankapuspi...),
> Vaira prash jelly to rejuvenate (main ingredients : Aswaganda, Bala...);

- **Correct routine of life**

Wake up early morning before six, attend to natural urgency, clean teeth mouth, tongue and treat the five senses using appropriated medicated oil. Use warm water in winter, cold water in summer.

Drink a glass of hot water or Niragada tisane.

Apply appropriate oil on head, feet, hands and have a shower.

Attend to your regular spiritual practices for twenty minutes.

An hour after the awakening have a light breakfast and start duties.

Have always lunch at midday, eating the food with satisfaction.

Have a light supper together with your family, talking about everyone's needs and thoughts.

Go to bed early, possibly at ten p. m. after the digestion. For at least half an hour before sleeping, avoid intellectually and emotionally heavy activities, do not have discussions, do not read nor watch violent films.

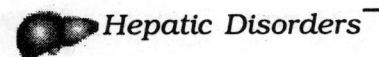

Hepatic Disorders
The NYM technique
I consider "NYM" an easy and very interesting instrument to create a balanced energy in subtle form for wellbeing. You may be curious about what "NYM" is. It is very simple and everyone could practice in his daily life, it needs about thirty minutes, and its aim is to bring harmony to the individual together with physical body, energy, intellect, emotion and destiny. The method is based on the individual date of birth and the feeling everyone has about his name. It is not astrology, nor even numerology, but a process of transcending the natural flow of life with pure consciousness.

Liver : the main filter
    As mother earth
    My experience

Liver – levels
    Physical :   from food to 5 elements
    Mental :   Perception of emotion
    Intellectual   management of food and emotion
    Spiritual toward overall harmony among other levels

Liver – disease : its origin is in the life style

Lack of harmony	Spiritual unbalance
Bad management of ego	Intellectual confusion
Block or over excitement	Emotional conflict
Food not digested according to body needs	Physical disorder

Treatment : life style correction
Modo di cura
Corpo, Sensi, Mente, Comportamento e Ambiente
Uso del consocenza
    Yoga
    Ayurveda
    Nome Yantra Mantra (NYM)

A reporter interviews a physician
How are you so excellent in diagnosis and treatment ? Is you the best in your family ? Ho, no ! My uncle is able to recognize before the beginning of illness. He is known by our family, only. And my father is able to recognize the illness at its very initial stage. He is known by many of our friends. And then I need the illness comes out to recognize it. Thus I am very well known ... I even went to cure the king and now I am having an interview ...

The common reason which lead the liver into disease are :
Alcolic drings

Hepatic Disorders

Havy meet
Chochllate
Drugs
Farmaci with colostral effect
Angry
Disappointment
Dislike

Incompatible food : food which contain equal amount of hot (acid) and cold (alkaline) energy. Cold energy food based on mainly starch which should not mixed with hot energy in equal amount, but could mixed very little amount.

Food better to eat one group at a time to avoid liver disorders.

Cold energy food : bread, wheat, rise, cerial, cakes, budin, oil, butter, cooked fruits, te, sweet

Hot energy food : meet, fish, milk, yogurt, formaggi, margerin, raw fruit, fruit drings, vine

To maintain the liver in health fellow :

Do not eat after one heavy discussion o angry
Do not have a heavy discussion while eating
Avoid cold food and drinks
Avoid drinking too much during the food
At the end of the meal have a hot digestive infusion
Have maximum satisfaction after meal
Yogasana
Meditation and Nadishuddhi ringuvnate the liver tissues.
Each Asana related with certain organ of the body by stimulating particular muscle

Natarajasana and Mayrasana by stimulating the muscles of petorali maggiori and deltoid protect the liver function.

When disorder in liver it is better practicing Patchimotasana which relax the liver by stimulating posterior thigh muscles.

NYM

NYM practices purify the liver in energetic levels and ricirculate the balanced energy flow.

Swami Joytimayananda
Joytinat Centre, VIABALBI 33/29, 16/29 GENOVA, GE, ITALY
TELE / FAX : 0039 0102758507, 0 0039 0102726422
EMAIL : Joytinat@mbox.ulisse.it

Hepatic Disorders

Importance Of Consideration Of Yakrut In The Treatment Of Sandhi Vikaras.

Vd. N. M. Pendse.

Brief outline

Yakrut is described as moolasthanam of Rakta Dhatu. Yakrut disorders cause vitiation of Rakta Dhatu. Hence, for proper formation and functioning of the Rakta Dhatu it is important to have a property functioning Yakrut.

The Rakta Dhatu performs various karmas (actions) which directly or indirectly control functioning of other dhatus / organs in the body.

Sandhi vikaras are important in view of their ability to cause deterioration of normal movements in an individual. They are also usually quite painful.

The causal relationship between vitiated Rakta Dhatu & Sandhi vikaras is emphasized in diseases like 'Vatrakta'

But, it's (Rakta Dhatu) consideration is of profound importance in the effective management of other Sandhi vikaras also.

This paper discusses the clinical observation & experiences of the above.

Vd. Narendra N. Pendse.
C-3/4, Yogayog Society, Bibwewadi, Pune 411 037.
Tel.: 020 421 3920 (R) 020 421 5650 (c)

Alcoholic Hepatitis

Dr. Shobhana J. Bhatia, Jaison Varghese

Introduction :

Alcoholic liver disease is a major complication of harmful alcohol use associated with a high morbidity and mortality. As in the western world in India also alcohol has emerged to be one of the leading causes of cirrhosis of liver. The spectrum of hepatic involvement spreads from asymptomatic fatty liver, alcoholic hepatitis to frank cirrhosis with decompensation. The course of the illness may be complicated by ascites, encephalopathy, variceal bleed, coagulopathy, spontaneous bacterial peritonitis and renal dysfunction. Each of the above mentioned complications being associated with a high morbidity and mortality.

Quantity of alcohol ingested (independent from the form in which it is ingested) is the single most important risk factor for the development of ALD. The minimum amount of alcohol intake associated with an increased risk for developing ALD ranged from 40 to 80 grams daily for 10 to 12 years.

One unit of alcohol contains 10-12 grams of alcohol which is equivalent to one ounce of spirits, twelve ounce of beer or four ounce glass of wine.

The three most widely recognised forms of alcoholic liver disease are alcoholic fatty liver (steatosis), acute alcoholic hepatitis, and alcoholic cirrhosis.

Grant et. Al. estimated that at least 80% of heavy drinkers show some features of fatty liver, 10-35% develop alcoholic hepatitis and approximately 10% develop cirrhosis.

Alcoholic hepatitis :

The average period of excessive drinking necessary for development of alcoholic hepatitis is approximately 15-20 years. While it is mostly a reversible condition, it my cause acute liver failure and portal hypertension. In severe alcoholic hepatitis, liver damage often increases

Hepatic Disorders

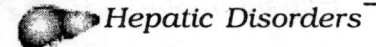

for 2-4 months after the patients admission to hospital despite abstinence and the condition may progress to hepatic failure and death during hospitalization.

Acute mortality rate have been reported to range from 13% in mild alcoholic hepatitis to 29-55% in severe cases. Nutritional status affects prognosis : A 30 day mortality rate of 2% is seen in patients with mild protein – energy malnutrition contrasts with one of 52% in those with severe protein energy malnutrition.

Women with alcoholic hepatitis are more likely to progress to cirrhosis than men.

According to Marbet 68% of patients with severe alcoholic hepatitis and 27% of patients with mild alcoholic hepatitis progressed to cirrhosis over a period of 4-8 years. When alcoholic hepatitis is superimposed on cirrhosis, the prognosis is particularly poor. A recent study showed that the 4 year survival rate decreased from 58% to 35% when alcoholic hepatitis was superimposed on cirrhosis. Nutrition : Protein energy malnutrition is present in 100% of patients with alcoholic hepatitis. Mendenhall et. aL. observed that PEM closely corelates with severity of alcoholic hepatitis, with or without cirrhosis and with mortality. One month mortality is 50% in severe PEM, and at one year it becomes 76%. Polyunsaturated fatty acids and dietary pork act as facilitating factor in high incidence of cirrhosis among alcoholics Saturated fatty acid and cholesterol appear to have a protective effect against cirrhosis.

Women are more susceptible than men to alcohol related liver disease, and are at greater risk of developing alcoholic hepatitis and cirrhosis. Women are more likely to develop cirrhosis at a younger age, at lower levels of alcohol consumption (exceeding 20 grams/day compared with over 40 grams / d for men), and after a shorter period of alcohol abuse (by approximately 6 years) than men.

In contrast to men, women are more likely to progress rapidly from alcoholic hepatitis to cirrhosis even after abstinence, and have reduced survival rate. Of women who continue to drink, only 30% survive 5 years compared to 76% of men. Women also tend to die at a younger age by approximately 8-12 years. It is more difficult to treat women with alcoholic liver disease and are likely candidates for relapse.

The increased vulnerability of women to alcohol induced liver injury has been attributed to the significantly higher blood alcohol concentrations, lower volume of distribution of alcohol due to higher proportion of fatty tissue, lower body size and a hormonal status different from men. In alcoholic women, the gastric mucosal alcohol dehydrogenase activity is lower than in men, and the first pass metabolism is virtually abolished leading to an increased bio-availability of alcohol.

Alcoholic Hepatitis (AH) :

AH (or steatohepatitis) has been estimated to occur in approximately 40% of chronic alcoholics. Histologically, the lesion occurs in the perivenular area. It comprises a constellation of changes, of which the essential features are (I) liver cell injury with ballooning and necrosis and often with Mallory bodies, (ii) an inflammatory cell – infiltrate, predominantly composed of neutrophil polymorphs, and (iii) pericellular fibrosis.

The cytoplasm of ballooned hepatocytes have a finely granular appearance producing a cobweb-like appearance. This ballooning degeneration is thought to be due to microtubule dysfunction with consequent impaired protein secretion accompanied by fluid retention. Ballooned hepatocytes may contain homogenous, eosinophilic, perinuclear inclusions, the Mallory bodies. Mallory bodies in AH comprises clusters of randomly oriented fibrils of 5 to 20 mm diameters.

The inflammatory infiltrate of AH is predominantly composed of neutrophil polymorphs which accumulate around necrotic liver cells and Mallory – bodies containing hepatocytes. Characteristically, the polymorphs surround the injured liver cells (satellitosis); the intensity of the infiltrate may be related to the number of Mallory bodies. There is evidence that they are chemotactic for neutrophils. Giant mitochondria may be observed within ballooned hepatocytes.

Fibrosis is an early and constant feature of alcoholic hepatitis. Individual hepatocytes or groups of hepatocytes become surrounded by fibrous tissue producing a so-called chicken – wire pattern. Although not pathognomonic, it is a highly characteristic feature. In addition to pericellular fibrosis there is often fibrous thickening around hepatic vein redicals, a process which has been refered to a phlebosclerosis.

Perivenular fibrosis (PF) :

Several groups have demonstrated that perivenular fibrosis, usually accompanied by pericellular fibrosis, may occur in the absence of hepatitis, that is in the absence, of inflammation, Mallory bodies or liver cell necrosis. In a study by Lieber's group identified patients with fatty liver and perivenular fibrosis, were at a greater risk of progression to irreversible liver disease than patients with fatty liver alone.

Maddrey's Index (Discriminant Function)

Discriminant function = [4.7 X Prothrombin time (s)] + Serum bilirubin (mg/dl)

OR

= [4.6 X (prothrombin time – control time) (s)] + serum bilirubin (mg / dl)

Hepatic Disorders

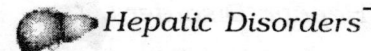

Discriminant function more than 93 using first formula and more than 32 in second formula or spontaneous hepatic encephalopathy predicted poor prognosis and high mortality. In patients with Maddrey's index > 32 treated with prednisolone 40 mg daily for 28 days, mortality at the end of treatment was 6% in steroid treated group which was significantly lower than in patients receiving the placebo preparations 35%.

As prognosis of cirrhosis depends on various factors, it is extremely important to use criteria which allow determination of prognosis in an individual patient with the best possible accuracy, especially during decision making for portacaval shunt surgery or liver transplantation. This ideal goal has not yet been reached, but several attempts have been made.

Historically the first of these attempts was made by Child and Turcotte to help select cirrhotic patients for portacaval shunt surgery. Several modifications of original Child and Turcotte classification have been proposed. The most used is that of Pugh et al.

Table : Paugh's grading for severity of liver disease.

Clinical & biochemical measurements	Points.		
	1	2	3
Encephalopathy	None	Mild	Severe
Ascites	None	Slight	Mod – severe
S. bilirubin (mg%)	< 2	2.3	> 3
S. Albumin (g/dl)	> 3.5	2.8 – 3.5	< 2.8
PT Difference (seconds)	< 4	4 – 6	> 6

They have omitted the assessment of body nutrition, included prothrombin time and made use of the weighting system whereby 1, 2 or 3 points are scored for increasing abnormality of each of the five 'variables' measured.

Addition of these values leads to modified Child's risk grades for each patients, points 5 & 6 – child A, 7 to 9 child B, 10 to 15 Child C.

The qualitites of simplicity, availability, low cost and good predictive power with regard to short term (1 year) survival, make the Pugh's score very useful. Poor prognosis is generally associated with low prothrombin index, marked ascites, gastrointestinal haemorrhage, advanced age, high daily alcohol consumption, serum bilirubin, serum alkaline phosphatase, low serum albumin, poor nutrition and presence of encephalopathy.

Hepatic Disorders

With still more complex models, large varices at endoscopy, high hepatic vein pressure gradient and low indocyanine green clearance were independently associated with a high risk of bleeding and a poor prognosis.

Child's class is inferior to a prognostic index based on multivariate analysis of prognostic factors 20. Other prognostic index has been used in particular clinical situations like, the Combined Clinical Laboratory Index (CCLI) of the University of Toronto 14 for alcoholic liver disease.

Pathogenesis of Alcoholic liver disease :

Redox Alteration : Ethanol metabolism in the liver is catalysed primarily by alcohol dehydrogenase (ADH) and cytochrome. Ethanol is metabolised to acetate, acetaldehyde being the intermediate compound. NADH accumulates during this metabolic process, which shifts the redox state of the hepatocytes. This ultimately affects the lipid and carbohydrate metabolism leading to hepatic steatosis and hypoglycemia respectively.

Oxidant Stress :

Alcohol metabolism via cytochrome PZEI pathway produces free radicals like hydroxy ethyl, superoxide and hydroxyl which damage intracellular organelles. Mitochondrial dysfunction caused by oxidant stress induced damage to mitohondrial DNA leads to microvesicular steatosis. Free radicals also cause hepatic lipid peroxidation and fibrosis.

Acetaldehyde Effect :

Acetaldehyde via the aldehyde oxidase and xanthine oxidase system generate free radicals. It also impairs mitochondrial beta oxidation. Acetaldehyde reacts with protein residue to form aldehyde protein adduct. This accumulates in the pericentral zone, where it mounts an immune response by acting as a neoantigen. The end result is ballooning of hepatocytes and stimulation of collagen synthesis.

Cytokines : Interleukins and TNF alpha are increased in alcoholic hepatitis. IL 8 is chemoattractant causing neutrophilic infiltration. IL 1, 6 and TNF produces direct liver injury. IL 6 and TGF B are responsible for hepatic fibrosis.

The above mentioned factors, activates the stellate cells to transform into myofibroblast like cell producing collagen. The end result is perisinusoidal fibrosis.

Clinical features of Alcoholic Hepatitis

Patients with severe alcoholic hepatitis are very ill and toxic. Usual modes of presentation are anorexia, nausea, vomiting, weakness, loose watery diarrhoea etc. Fever upto 40'C may be present in 75% patients. On general examination jaundice, spider naevi and palmar erythema can be noticed. Hepatomegaly is present in more than 75% of patients, spleen being palpable in 5-10%. Patient can have associated ascites, hepatic encephalopathy and gastrointestinal bleed.

Hepatic Disorders

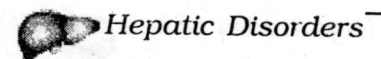

Laboratory Investigations :

Macrocytic anemia is present in 75% of patients due to reduced folate and vitamin B and C levels and bone marrow depression. AST and ALT levels are elevated but rarely exceeds more than 300 U/L. AST/ALT is more than 2 because pyridoxine deficiency affects ALT more than ALT. Serum gamma glutamyl transferase is elevated in 60% of alcoholics consuming more than 80 grams of alcohol per day.

Test of recent alcohol consumption

The levels of mitochondrial AST, serum carbohydrate deficient transferrin, antibody against acetaldehyde protein adducts, collagen polypeptides and laminin are used to test for recent alcohol consumption.

Complications of Alcoholic hepatitis :

Complications are similar to other chronic liver disease namely encephalopathy, coagulopathy, hepato-renal syndrome, gastrointestinal haemorrhage, ascites and infections.

Medical Management :

Abstinence : Abstinence is the cornerstone of treatment for alcoholic liver disease. Abstinence improves the liver histology, reduces the portal hypertension and decreases the chances of progression to cirrhosis.

Nutritional therapy : Protein energy malnutrition of varying severity is prevalent in almost 100% of patients with alcoholic hepatitis. Quality nutrition with proteins one gram per kilogram body weight and a minimum of 30 K Calories per kilogram body weight improves the liver histology, liver function tests and the Child score. All the investigators except Narrallah could not demonstrate any survival benefit with improved nutrition.

Enteral feeding is the best if the patient can tolerate, peripheral parenteral nutrition being the next choice, total parenteral nutrition being the last choice. Branched chain amino acids supplements precipitate hepatic encephalopathy.

Water and electrolyte balance should be monitored and managed accordingly.

Corticosteroids :

Steroids suppress the immune response, decrease the fibrotic activity in the liver and improves the appetite and well being on the patient. There are thirteen randomised controlled trials and three meta analysis on the effect of steroid on mortality in alcoholic hepatitis. Patients with gastrointestinal bleed were excluded from most of the trials. Carithers et. al. selected patients with discriminant function more than 32 or spontaneous hepatic enephalopathy for steroid therapy and demonstrated significant survival benefit at twenty-eight days. A meta-analysis by Christensen which included twelve trials did not show any significant survival benefit.

Others treatment options tried in the past are anabolic steroids, propyl thiouracil, colchicine, malotilate, cyanidanol, silymarins, penicillamine, pentoxiphylline, ursodeoxycholic acid and insiulin plus glucagon therapy. None of these were shown to be of any benefit.

Liver transplantation

Patient with end stage alcoholic liver disease do as well as non – alcoholic liver disease after transplantation. Patients who are child C without any extra hepatic organ damage who are abstaining for more than six months can be offered liver transplantation with good result.

Data on patients with alcoholic hepatitis

Profile of alcoholic hepatitis in Mumbai. Jaison Verghese, Amitabh S. Naik, Sundeep S. Shah, Shobna J. Bhatia, Vinod Krishnaradha, Mangal Kate. Department of Gastroenterology, TN Medical College and BYL Nair Hospital, Mumbai – 400 008. Background :- Alcoholic hepatitis is a serious complication of alcohol abuse.

Aims and Methods : To find out the clinical and biochemical features of associated hepatitis, 127 patients with alcoholic liver disease seen over the last 1 year were evaluated. Patients who had features of alcoholic hepatitis : raised AST (> 80 IU/L) and / or raised bilirubin (> 5 mg%) were included in the study.

Results : Seventy three patients (mean age 45.5 [SD 10.2] y; 65 men) had alcoholic hepatitis. The duration and quantity of alcohol consumption were 17.2 (7) y and 212.7 (83) g/day, respectively. The clinical features on presentation were jaundice (n=67), ascites (64), gastrointestinal bleed (29), encephalopathy (31), coagulaopathy (2), palmar erythema (35), spider nevi (50), gynecomastia (29) and testicular atrophy (10). The duration of illness was 3.8 (6.5) months; median 2 months. Biochemical parameters were total bilirubin 12.8 (8.1) mg%, (direct bilirubin 8.6 [5.5]), total proteins 5.5 (0.8) g/dL (albumin 2.4 [0.5]), alkaline phosphatase 4.9 (5.9) BU, AST 111 (62) IU, ALT 64.9 (92.5) IU, AST/ALT ratio 2.6 (1.1), prothrombin time 18.7 (4.8) s (control 11). BUN 20.3 (17.4) mg/dl, serum creatinine 1 (0.69) mg/dL, serum sodium 127.8 (8.2) meq/l, urinary sodium 45.5 (26.6) meq/l, Child-Pughs class; B 11, C 62. Maddrey's index 47.2 (26); the index was >32 in 53 patients. Mean creatinine clearance was 43.7 (31.3) mL/min; creatinine clearance was <40 mL/min in 24 (33%) patients at presentation. Ascitic fluid protenis 0.54 g/dl. Viral markers for HBs Ag and anti-HCV were positive in 7 and 3 cases, respectively; HIV was positive in one patient. At one month, 27 (37%) patients died of progressive renal failure, worsening liver function, encephalopathy or bleed. In patients who survived, the bilirubin, BUN, creatinine, Maddrey's index were significantly lower, and albumin and serum sodium levels were significantly higher.

Conclusions:

A significant proportion of patients with chronic alcoholic liver disease have associated hepatitis. Almost one-third have renal dysfunction and the mortality at one month is 37%.

Various Management of Rudhapath Kamala (Obstructive Jaundice

Vd. Anant Dharmadhikari

"Ruddhapatha Kamala" is described along with Panduroga in Charaka Samhita. Symptoms of this type of KAMALA can be correlated with "viral Hepatitis" for treating the same, commonly used drug is Arogyavardhini & punarnavashtaka Kwath

Some factors compel us to think for the alternative for Arogyavardhini viz.

i) Unavailability of Arogyavardhini

ii) Doubtful or short time preparation methods of kalpa

In this condition the physician has to select a drug having some specific criterias.

This paper discusses the same.

The procedure of selecting alternative drug substance or drug is explained in Ayurvedic texts.

1. If the drug substance or drug belong to specific group & its not available then the other drugs available in the same group can be considered. Also

न शास्त्रमात्र शरणं गच्छेत नचालोचिताभय:

By studying the exact qualities of a drug the other drug having same properties

In any disease drug selection guideline is

एवं अन्यान् अविव्याधीन् स्वनिदान विपर्यात् ।

चिकित्सेन् अनुबंधेत्सु सति हेतु विपर्ययस् ।

Hepatic Disorders

त्यक्त्वा यथायथं दैद्यो युंजात् व्याधिविपर्ययम् । अ.सू. ८/२२,२३

टीका संतर्पणोत्थो अपतर्पणेन

शीतात्थो - उष्णेन इत्यादी

'Nidan Viparita Chikiitsa' **is the main principle.**

If the disease persist for longer time or recover then the hetu viparyaya chikitsa should be given up & vyadhi viparita chikitsa should be adopted,

Hetu / Nidana Viparita means –

Absence of Hetu properties & actions opposite to dosas (which are increased by hetu) = mainly shodhana.

The Rudhapatha Kamala is Kaphaj vyadhi i.e. dominance of kapha in the samprapti.

Considering hetu, prolonged or continuous consumption of haphazard diet or action is important.

The same disease is santarpavajanye.

So consider the hetu responsible for this disease, e.g.

The points has daily routine since 3-4 years

After waking up in the morning he drinks water – 500ml	6.00 O'clock
Tea, bread / biscuits	7.00 O'clock
No exercise,	
1 glass milk + 1 egg or 1 chappati	9.00 O'clock
In the office - Idali, Kachori	11.00 O'clock
Lunch (containing curd 1 bowl)	
After meal 1 fruit immediately + water 1 lt.	1.00 O'clock
Lassi / Pepsi	5.00 O'clock
Evening – fruit juice 1 glass	6.00 O'clock
Dinner + 1 lt. Water	9.00 O'clock
Bed time 1 glass milk	11.00 O'clock

The main thing is Adhyashama & continuity in that.

So there is provocation of kapha & increase in the qualities like Drava Snigdha (unctuous), guru (heavy), manda (slow).

Hepatic Disorders

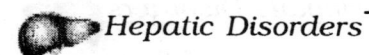

Hence the disease – Rudhapatha Kamala.

Principal of

Treatment concerned will be –

- To stop these 'Hetusevana' substances c

- Properties ushna, teekshna, rooksha which are opposite to above hetusevana should be administered. e.g. Rasa like Amla, Katu, Lavanva

Charaka has advised Trikatu Churna c Mastulunga Rasa, which have above properties

Also the diet should have the same properties e.g. Katu Amla Rasa Kuldtha

So we can consider any appropriate kalpa by studying all aspects of hetu viparita chikitsa.

Vd. Anant Dharmadhikari.
Poddar Ayurved Mahavidyalaya,, Vorli, Mumbai 400018.

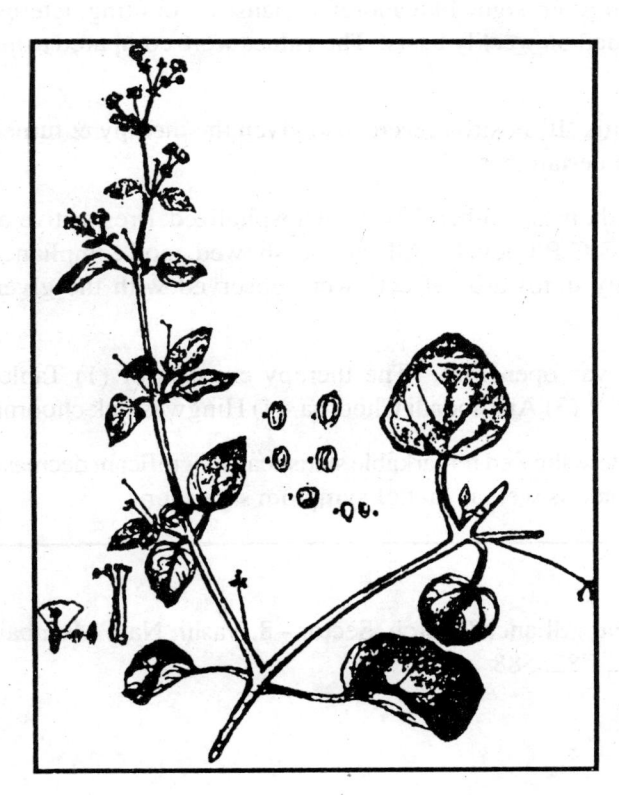

Sanskrit Name : Punarnava
Latin Name : Boerhavia diffusa

A Clinical Evaluation of an Ayurvedic Herbomineral Therapy in the Management of 120 Cases of Viral Hepatitis

Aashish S. Phadke

---

120 cases of viral hepatitis were studied, at Centre for Ayurved & Panchakarma Therapy, Navi Mumbai. All Patients were screened for their biochemical parameters such as Sr.Bilirubin, S.G.O.T., S.G.P.T. on 0-day, 7th day & 14th day & 21st day. Symptom - sign score specially prepared based on symptom-signs like anorexia, nausea, vomiting, icterus, filling general weakness & was recorded on weekly basis. The values were compared using appropriate statistical tool.

One patient found out to be Hepatitis 'B' positive, were also given the therapy & turned out to be Hepatitis 'B' negative, after certain period.

No patients were given modern medicines, neither they were hospitalized, irrespective of their very high values of Sr.Bilirubin, S.G.P.T. levels. All patients showed good compliance towards the therapy offered. No any untowards effects were observed with the given therapy.

A model used for clinical study was open trial. The therapy consists of (1) Tablet Arogyavardhini Rasa (2) Capsule Eld-1 (3) Ajamodadi Choorna. (4) Hingwashtak choorna

Majority of the patients except very few showed remarkable statistically significant decrease in their values of biochemical parameter as well as that of symptom sign score.

Dr.Aashish S.Phadke
Res. RH-1/B3, Sagar Vihar Road, Near Alliance Church, Sector - 8, Vashi, Navi Mumbai, Pin - 400 703, India. Tel. No. Res. 022-7823588